Development of a Surgeon: Medical School through Retirement

Editors

RONALD F. MARTIN
PAUL J. SCHENARTS

SURGICAL CLINICS
OF NORTH AMERICA

www.surgical.theclinics.com

Consulting Editor
RONALD F. MARTIN

February 2016 • Volume 96 • Number 1

ELSEVIER

1600 John F. Kennedy Boulevard • Suite 1800 • Philadelphia, Pennsylvania, 19103-2899

http://www.surgical.theclinics.com

SURGICAL CLINICS OF NORTH AMERICA Volume 96, Number 1
February 2016 ISSN 0039–6109, ISBN-13: 978-0-323-41714-3

Editor: John Vassallo, j.vassallo@elsevier.com
Developmental Editor: Colleen Viola

Surgical Clinics of North America (ISSN 0039–6109) is published bimonthly by Elsevier Inc., 360 Park Avenue South, New York, NY 10010-1710. Months of publication are February, April, June, August, October, and December. Business and Editorial Offices: 1600 John F. Kennedy Blvd., Suite 1800, Philadelphia, PA 19103-2899. Periodicals postage paid at New York, NY and additional mailing offices. Subscription prices are $375.00 per year for US individuals, $707.00 per year for US institutions, $100.00 per year for US students and residents, $455.00 per year for Canadian individuals, $895.00 per year for Canadian institutions, $510.00 for international individuals, $895.00 per year for international institutions and $250.00 per year for Canadian and foreign students/residents. To receive student/resident rate, orders must be accompanied by name of affiliated institution, date of term, and the *signature* of program/residency coordinator on institution letterhead. Orders will be billed at individual rate until proof of status is received. Foreign air speed delivery is included in all *Clinics* subscription prices. All prices are subject to change without notice. POSTMASTER: Send address changes to *Surgical Clinics*, Elsevier Health Sciences Division, Subscription Customer Service, 3251 Riverport Lane, Maryland Heights, MO 63043. **Customer Service (orders, claims, online, change of address): Telephone: 1-800-654-2452 (U.S. and Canada); 314-447-8871 (outside U.S. and Canada). Fax: 314-447-8029. E-mail: journalscustomerservice-usa@elsevier.com (for print support); journalsonline support-usa@elsevier.com (for online support).**

Reprints. For copies of 100 or more, of articles in this publication, please contact the Commercial Reprints Department, Elsevier Inc., 360 Park Avenue South, New York, New York 10010-1710. Tel. 212-633-3874, Fax: 212-633-3820, E-mail: reprints@elsevier.com.

The Surgical Clinics of North America is also published in Spanish by McGraw-Hill Interamericana Editores S.A., P.O. Box 5-237 06500 Mexico D.F. Mexico; and in Portuguese by Interlivros Edicoes Ltda., Rua Comandante Coelho 1085, CEP 21250, Rio de Janeiro, Brazil; and in Greek by Paschalidis Medical Publications, Athens Greece.

The Surgical Clinics of North America is covered in *MEDLINE/PubMed (Index Medicus)*, *EMBASE/Excerpta Medica*, *Current Contents/Clinical Medicine*, *Current Contents/Life Sciences*, *Science Citation Index*, and *ISI/BIOMED*.

Contributors

CONSULTING EDITOR

RONALD F. MARTIN, MD, FACS
Director of Surgical Education, Marshfield Clinic and Saint Joseph's Hospital, Marshfield, Wisconsin; Clinical Adjunct Professor of Surgery, University of Wisconsin School of Medicine and Public Health, Madison, Wisconsin; Colonel (ret.), United States Army Reserve, Medical Corps

EDITORS

RONALD F. MARTIN, MD, FACS
Director of Surgical Education, Marshfield Clinic and Saint Joseph's Hospital, Marshfield, Wisconsin; Clinical Adjunct Professor of Surgery, University of Wisconsin School of Medicine and Public Health, Madison, Wisconsin; Colonel (ret.), United States Army Reserve, Medical Corps

PAUL J. SCHENARTS, MD, FACS
Professor and Vice Chair of Academic Affairs, Chief of Trauma, Critical Care, Emergency Surgery, and Acute Care Surgery, Department of Surgery, University of Nebraska, College of Medicine, Omaha, Nebraska

AUTHORS

CHANDRAKANTH ARE, MD, MBA, FRCS, FACS
Jerald L and Carolynn J Varner Professor in Surgical Oncology and Global Health, Vice Chair Education, Program Director General Surgery Residency, University of Nebraska Medical Center, Omaha, Nebraska

PATRICE GABLER BLAIR, MPH
Associate Director, Division of Education, American College of Surgeons, Chicago, Illinois

JO BUYSKE, MD
Associate Executive Director and Director of Evaluation, American Board of Surgery; Adjunct Professor of Surgery, University of Pennsylvania School of Medicine, Philadelphia, Pennsylvania

SAMUEL CEMAJ, MD, FACS
Department of Surgery, University of Nebraska, College of Medicine, Omaha, Nebraska

THOMAS H. COGBILL, MD, FACS
Attending Surgeon, Department of General and Vascular Surgery, Gundersen Health System, La Crosse, Wisconsin

CHARITY H. EVANS, MD, MHCM
Assistant Professor, Department of Surgery, University of Nebraska Medical Center, Omaha, Nebraska

BRANDON T. GROVER, DO, FACS
Department of General and Vascular Surgery, Gundersen Health System, La Crosse, Wisconsin

REBECCA L. HOFFMAN, MD
Measey Education Resident Research Fellow, Department of Surgery, Perelman School of Medicine at the University of Pennsylvania, Philadelphia, Pennsylvania

JEREMIAH JONES, MD
Department of Surgical Education, Iowa Methodist Medical Center, Des Moines, Iowa

RACHEL R. KELZ, MD, MSCE
Associate Program Director, General Surgery Residency Program, Associate Professor, Department of Surgery, Perelman School of Medicine at the University of Pennsylvania, Philadelphia, Pennsylvania

SHANU N. KOTHARI, MD, FACS
Department of General and Vascular Surgery, Gundersen Health System, La Crosse, Wisconsin

LINDA K. LUPI, MBA
Senior Manager, Educational Administration and Special Programs, Division of Education, American College of Surgeons, Chicago, Illinois

RONALD F. MARTIN, MD, FACS
Director of Surgical Education, Marshfield Clinic and Saint Joseph's Hospital, Marshfield, Wisconsin; Clinical Adjunct Professor of Surgery, University of Wisconsin School of Medicine and Public Health, Madison, Wisconsin; Colonel (ret.), United States Army Reserve, Medical Corps

REBECCA M. MINTER, MD
Professor of Surgery; Alvin Baldwin Jr., Chair in Surgery; Vice Chair, Clinical Operations, Department of Surgery; Chief, Section of Hepatopancreatobiliary and GI Oncology; University of Texas Southwestern Medical Center, Dallas, Texas

JON B. MORRIS, MD
The Ernest F. Rosato-William Measey Professor in Surgical Education, Vice Chair for Education, Program Director, General Surgery Residency Program, Department of Surgery, Perelman School of Medicine at the University of Pennsylvania, Philadelphia, Pennsylvania

JOHN R. POTTS III, MD
Senior Vice President, Surgical Accreditation, ACGME, Chicago, Illinois; Adjunct Professor of Surgery, University of Texas Houston Medical School, Houston, Texas; Senior Scholar, Department of Medical Education, University of Illinois College of Medicine - Chicago, Chicago, Illinois

AJIT K. SACHDEVA, MD, FRCSC, FACS
Director, Division of Education, American College of Surgeons, Chicago, Illinois

CHRISTOPHER P. SCALLY, MD
Department of Surgery, University of Michigan, Ann Arbor, Michigan

KIMBERLY D. SCHENARTS, PhD
Professor, Department of Surgery, University of Nebraska Medical Center, Omaha, Nebraska

PAUL J. SCHENARTS, MD, FACS
Professor and Vice Chair of Academic Affairs, Chief of Trauma, Critical Care, Emergency Surgery, and Acute Care Surgery, Department of Surgery, University of Nebraska, College of Medicine, Omaha, Nebraska

KERI SEYMOUR, DO
Assistant Professor, Department of Surgery, Duke University Medical Center, Durham, North Carolina

STEPHEN B. SHAPIRO, MD, FACS
Attending Surgeon, Department of General and Vascular Surgery, Gundersen Health System, La Crosse, Wisconsin

RICHARD A. SIDWELL, MD
Program Director of General Surgery Residency, Department of Surgical Education, Iowa Methodist Medical Center, Des Moines, Iowa; Adjunct Clinical Professor, Department of Surgery, University of Iowa Carver College of Medicine, Iowa City, Iowa

RANJAN SUDAN, MD
Associate Professor, Department of Surgery, Duke University Medical Center, Durham, North Carolina

Contents

This review outlines the current state of undergraduate medical education for the surgeon in training and highlights ongoing efforts to improve the preparation of graduating students entering surgical residency. Possible models for improved integration of specialty specific training in medical school are explored, and future directions in undergraduate surgical education are considered in the context of ongoing curricular initiatives in medical schools within North America.

Competency is an individual trait. As an agency that accredits programs and institutions, the Accreditation Council for Graduate Medical Education (ACGME) does not define or access competency. However, in the past 15 years the ACGME has promulgated several initiatives to aid programs in the assessment of the competence of their residents and fellows. Those initiatives include the Outcomes Project (which codified the competencies), the Milestones, and the Clinical Learning Environment Review Program. In the near future, the ACGME will implement an initiative by which programs can develop and study the results of competency-based residency curricula.

Surgical training graduates require a period of adjustment as they transform from trainees to experienced surgeons. Making a smooth transition is important for patient safety and new surgeon success. A subset of current graduates does not feel confident to enter directly into practice. Residency design with curriculum refocus, credentialing to encourage graded responsibility, and increased operative exposure is necessary. Onboarding programs should include formal mentoring, career counseling, proctoring by senior surgeons, and objective review of outcomes. The ACS developed a one-year TTP program to provide independent decision-making, operative autonomy, mentoring by senior surgeons, and practice management experience.

Since the late 1880s, surgical residency programs have existed in forms that are similar to our current models. Many important variations have been introduced over time. On aggregate this system has worked remarkably well; though as economic, demographic, and cultural changes continue to evolve, one must wonder if we were to change our models, how might we do that and what reasoning could we use. This article's focus is to take a stratospheric view of what could be done, particularly in the United States, rather than characterize what happens in other countries with other health economic systems.

Surgical subspecialties are now well-established, and many surgery residents pursue fellowship training for various reasons. Fellowships can bridge the gaps found in many residency programs by providing graduating residents with opportunities to master surgical skills, gain confidence and progressive autonomy, and receive further mentorship. The experience also eases the transition to independent practice by allowing surgeons to tailor their training to coincide with personal interests and future practice goals. It is unlikely that the number of surgery residents pursuing fellowship training will decrease, so it is important to provide the infrastructure, oversight, and opportunities to meet their needs.

The past two decades have been witness to some of the most dynamic changes that have occurred in surgical education in all of its history. Political policies, social revolution, and the competing priorities of a new generation of surgical trainees are defining the needs of modern training paradigms. Although the university-based academic program's tripartite mission of clinical service, research, and education has remained steadfast, the mechanisms for achieving success in this mission necessitate adaptation and innovation. The resource-rich learning environment and the unique challenges that face university-based programs contribute to its ability to generate the future leaders of the surgical workforce.

Training competent and professional surgeons efficiently and effectively requires innovation and modernization of educational methods. Today's medical learner is quite adept at using multiple platforms to gain information, providing surgical educators with numerous innovative avenues to promote learning. With the growth of technology, and the restriction of work hours in surgical education, there has been an increase in use of simulation, including virtual reality, robotics, telemedicine, and gaming. The use of simulation has shifted the learning of basic surgical skills to

the laboratory, reserving limited time in the operating room for the acquisition of complex surgical skills.

Ranjan Sudan and Keri Seymour

Impaired physicians are unable to manage professional activities safely.
Impairment can be the result of physical or mental disorders, but impaired
physicians commonly refers to those suffering from substance use disorders. These disorders are at least as common in physicians as they are in
the general population, and physician health programs have been established in each state to provide expeditious and detailed evaluation, referral
to treatment facilities, and post-treatment monitoring to ensure compliance. These programs protect participants against sanctions and safe-
guard patients. The prognosis for participants is excellent, with more
than 70% able to practice medicine at 5 years.

Chandrakanth Are

The health care environment in the United States is witnessing major
changes. The Halstedian model has produced surgeons who joined the
workforce for over a century. While the Halstedian model will continue to
be of benefit, we need to be proactive and develop innovative models of
graduate medical education that meet the needs of the 21st century.
The history of graduate medical education is punctuated by surgical
leaders that made great contributions. The time is ripe again for the surgical community to develop innovative models of graduate medical education that will continue to sustain the surgical workforce of the future.

Ajit K. Sachdeva, Patrice Gabler Blair, and Linda K. Lupi

Surgeons have specific education and training needs as they enter practice, progress through the core period of active practice, and then as
they wind down their clinical work before retirement. These transitions
and the career progression process, combined with the dynamic health
care environment, present specific opportunities for innovative education
and training based on practice-based learning and improvement and
continuous professional development methods. Cutting-edge technologies, blended models, simulation, mentoring, preceptoring, and integrated
approaches can play critical roles in supporting surgeons as they provide
the best surgical care throughout various phases of their careers.

Paul J. Schenarts and Samuel Cemaj

Surgeons suffer from the same physiologic impairments common to all
people with advancing age. These impairments not only affect the surgeon
but also the patients under their care. This article delineates the epidemiologic context of the graying population of surgeons and the cognitive and

physiologic changes that occur as the result of aging, the consequence of which is that greater experience does not necessarily equate with better clinical outcomes. This work also addresses potential methods for the ongoing evaluation of the aging surgeon and how elder surgeons may be best used as they reach the conclusion of their career.

Surgical learning starts in medical school and continues through retirement. Assessment of knowledge and skills across a variety of arenas at each stage is an obligation of the profession in its duty to the public. The American Board of Surgery is engaged in standardization and assessment to a greater or lesser degree at each stage of surgical learning.

Independent academic medical centers have been training surgeons for more than a century; this environment is distinct from university or military programs. There are several advantages to training at a community program, including a supportive learning environment with camaraderie between residents and faculty, early and broad operative experience, and improved graduate confidence. Community programs also face challenges, such as resident recruitment and faculty engagement. With the workforce needs for general surgeons, independent training programs will continue to play an integral role.

SURGICAL CLINICS
OF NORTH AMERICA

ISSUE OF RELATED INTEREST

Anesthesiology Clinics, December 2015 (Vol. 33, Issue 4)
Value-Based Care
Lee A. Fleisher, *Editor*
Available at: www.anesthesiology.theclinics.com

THE CLINICS ARE AVAILABLE ONLINE!
Access your subscription at:
www.theclinics.com

Foreword

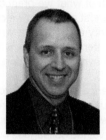

Ronald F. Martin, MD, FACS
Consulting Editor

In many of the forewords to previous issues of the *Surgical Clinics of North America*, we have discussed that part of the ongoing mission is to explore those topics that define general surgery. I have also written about how elusive it can be to identify what really constitutes general surgery or, for that matter, what makes a general surgeon a general surgeon. In past issues, we have wrestled with the balance of generalization and specialization, practice in highly populated areas versus rural or austere environments, even routine environments versus war environments or systems compromised by natural disaster. While those concepts are all of great importance, we are putting them aside for the moment so that we may consider a topic that is absolutely of common interest by addressing one immutable fact of being a surgeon: we train, we practice, and we eventually stop working. It doesn't really matter what exactly we do along the way, we all follow the same basic arc.

In past issues, we have addressed surgical education, workforce issues, regulatory and certification topics, as well as others in various contexts either separately or combined with other topics. In this issue, we have made a conscious decision to look at the entire path a surgeon follows from medical school through retirement as well as to discuss the various milestone options, such as fellowship training, board certification, and maintenance of certification requirements one encounters along the way. These are common to nearly everyone, and I am fairly certain everyone has an opinion about these commonalities.

One of the privileges of being the Consulting Editor for the series is that I arrange the topics for the issues and get to invite the Guest Editors; occasionally I serve as a Guest Editor or Co-Guest Editor as well. For this issue, I reached out to Dr P.J. Schenarts to work with me on this topic. I asked Dr Schenarts for his help for many reasons. To begin with, P.J. has an unparalleled passion for education and a limitless willingness to consider all sides of an issue. Dr Schenarts and I were surgical residents together many years ago, and we were both trained very much to question everything and push ourselves to every limit. Even though I was only a few years ahead of P.J. in training, he has always had a better intuitive sense of the newer generation of surgical trainees than I ever possessed. I was confident that P.J. would push me as well as the rest of our collaborators on every topic in this issue as well—and he did not disappoint me.

Surg Clin N Am 96 (2016) xiii–xiv
http://dx.doi.org/10.1016/j.suc.2015.10.003
0039-6109/16/$ – see front matter © 2016 Published by Elsevier Inc.

surgical.theclinics.com

We reached out to the best people in the very best positions we could think of for their views and insights into each topic, and we specifically wanted divergent and even potentially oppositional views on these topics. While much of what we practice as surgeons is grounded in the best hard science we can find, almost all of what we do to train ourselves and follow our career paths is rooted in history and tradition with perhaps a little science thrown in. In our opinion, providing alternative views was not a nicety but a necessity for this issue. To that end, we have also considered how things might look if we started from scratch.

As always, we strive to make the *Surgical Clinics of North America* not only a source of information but also a basis for discussion and further thought—this issue is no different. For this issue specifically, we went to a well of people who are under tremendous demands for their time and efforts. All of them are not only valued colleagues but also valued friends. One would be very hard pressed to find anybody in a better position to give her or his views than the group we assembled. The series is deeply indebted to all the contributors to this issue, who gave generously of their time and effort when most of them had little to no extra of either to give so that we may be better positioned to consider how our profession should maintain and replicate itself as we go forth.

As with all issues of the *Surgical Clinics of North America*, we look forward to your feedback as well. As I stated earlier, we desire a dialogue. In the meanwhile, I trust you will find much in this issue that will give you something to reflect on or reminisce about, perhaps even to reject. We are all in the profession of serving our communities, and we are all responsible for making sure our profession is left in better stead than we found it. I hope this issue will give you a platform to base your improvements.

Ronald F. Martin, MD, FACS
Marshfield Clinic
Saint Joseph's Hospital
University of Wisconsin School
of Medicine and Public Health
1000 North Oak Avenue
Marshfield, WI 54449, USA

E-mail address:
rmartin@yorkhospital.com

Preface

Development of a Surgeon

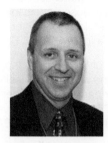 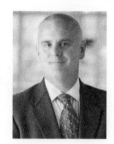

Ronald F. Martin, MD, FACS   Paul J. Schenarts, MD, FACS
Editors

The Canadian philosopher, Herbert Marshall McLuhan, once said, "Innumerable confusions and a feeling of despair invariably emerge in periods of great techno-logic and cultural transition." Clearly medicine in general and surgery in specific have been undergoing a monumental transition for more than a decade. At first blush, evolution over this timeframe may appear slow. Given our proud surgical his-tory and entrenched traditions, however, this evolution has been at a supersonic pace. As a result, surgeons in practice and those charged with training the next generations have felt a sense of unease. The rise of the electronic medical record, our improved understanding of diseases, evolving technology, an aging and more complex patient population, as well as new requirements to remain in practice, have all coalesced into a nearly palpable sense of apprehension that can be felt across the full spectrum of practice. From the white-coat ceremonies for first-year medical students to retirement parties of surgeons leaving practice, how a surgeon should navigate their career is a constant and at times a vigorous discussion.

In this issue of *Surgical Clinics of North America*, we have gathered the opinions of some of the most prominent thought leaders in American Surgery to explore the devel-opment of a surgeon from medical school through retirement. The contributing authors represent a true cross-section of the surgical profession. This issue is particularly note-worthy, in that some authors outwardly disagree with other authors. This dichotomy was intentional and by design. It is only through such contradiction that real knowledge can evolve.

In closing, we would like to thank each of our fellow authors for their thoughtful and critical analysis of their assigned topics. As one might say, each of these authors is a

Surg Clin N Am 96 (2016) xv–xvi
http://dx.doi.org/10.1016/j.suc.2015.10.002
surgical.theclinics.com
0039-6109/16/$ – see front matter © 2016 Published by Elsevier Inc.

"heavy hitter." As such, we are greatly indebted to each for the time they invested into this project.

Ronald F. Martin, MD, FACS
Marshfield Clinic
Saint Joseph's Hospital
1000 North Oak Avenue
Marshfield, WI 54449, USA

University of Wisconsin School
of Medicine and Public Health
Department of Surgery
750 Highland Avenue
Madison, WI 53726, USA

Paul J. Schenarts, MD, FACS
Critical Care and Emergency Surgery
Department of Surgery
University of Nebraska
College of Medicine
983280 Nebraska Medical Center
Omaha, NE 68198-3280, USA

E-mail addresses:
rmartin@yorkhospital.com (R.F. Martin)
paul.schenarts@unmc.edu (P.J. Schenarts)

Medical School Training for the Surgeon

Christopher P. Scally, MD[a], Rebecca M. Minter, MD[b],*

KEYWORDS

- Medical education • Surgery resident prep curriculum
- Entrustable professional activities

KEY POINTS

- Currently, there is heterogeneity among graduating medical students in terms of their preparation for a surgery residency.
- Within undergraduate medical education, there is an ongoing paradigm shift from a broad-based, one-size-fits-all curriculum, to more focused preparation for future practice and residency specialty.
- Surgeons and medical educators must invest in developing integrated longitudinal programs to develop surgical trainees, beginning with medical school.

Surgery training is typically viewed as beginning July 1st, when new interns begin their surgery residency. The July intern is considered relatively undifferentiated, and attention within the surgical community has focused most often on the eventual development of that intern into a fully capable, trained surgeon over the course of a surgery residency. However, this traditional paradigm of focusing primarily on training during residency requires that medical school graduates enter residency training with adequate background medical knowledge, rudimentary but sound fundamental technical skills, and an understanding of the field and their role as junior residents. Recently, concerns have been raised regarding the heterogeneity of graduating students' readiness to take on these tasks, and a feeling that the first months of residency are often spent preparing newly minted residents to safely take the reins as a postgraduate year (PGY)1 resident. Moving forward, greater attention is needed to ensure our medical school graduates are optimally equipped to succeed, and that they enter

Funding: Dr Scally is supported by a grant from the National Cancer Institute (5T32CA009672-23). The views expressed herein do not necessarily represent the views of the United States Government.
Disclosures: None.
[a] Department of Surgery, University of Michigan, 1500 E. Medical Center Drive, Ann Arbor, MI 48109-5343, USA; [b] Department of Surgery, University of Texas Southwestern Medical Center, 5323 Harry Hines Boulevard, Dallas, TX 75390-9031, USA
* Corresponding author.
E-mail address: Rebecca.Minter@UTSouthwestern.edu

residency with a more cohesive skills set focused on the foundational abilities needed on the first day of their postgraduate training program.

This article outlines the current state of surgery training in undergraduate medical education. We also highlight ongoing efforts to improve the preparation of graduating students for Surgery residency, and to better incorporate specialty-specific surgery training within medical school. Finally, we focus on future directions in undergraduate surgical education, particularly taking into consideration ongoing curricular initiatives in medical schools across the United States.

SURGERY TRAINING IN THE TRADITIONAL MEDICAL SCHOOL CURRICULUM

The majority of students' surgery-specific training has traditionally occurred within the third year core clerkship and fourth year elective or subinternship rotations. However, surgery educators have raised concerns that these experiences are variable in terms of quality and duration of exposure, and that as a result, new interns are not prepared uniformly to begin their surgical residencies.[1-3]

A number of factors contribute to the variability in graduates' readiness for surgery training. Within the third year clerkship, medical schools vary widely in terms of how well students are incorporated into patient care and decision making. Further heterogeneity is introduced based on the clinical rotations to which students are assigned, with some medical schools having rotations predominantly in tertiary referral centers on services directed by highly specialized practitioners with focused practices, and other schools' rotations using community-based preceptors with broader general surgery practices. Beyond this variability within the third year clerkship rotations, schools and students vary widely in their approach to the fourth year of medical school. Rotations include electives of various rigor, subinternships, and the increasingly common visiting audition rotations at outside institutions.[4]

In addition to this variation in exposure, concerns have been raised that medical students are increasingly marginalized during their clinical rotations, and clinical clerkships more closely resemble "observerships" with less active roles for students. Although the electronic medical record has a number of advantages for patient care and ease of accessing information, the implementation of many of these systems have limited students' ability to participate in clinical documentation.[5] Many graduates have little experience writing traditional history and physical examinations, brief operative notes, daily progress notes, and discharge summaries. The loss of this active experience negatively impacts their efficiency with these tasks as they enter residency. A number of invested parties, including the Association of American Medical Colleges (AAMC), the American Medical Association, and the Carnegie Foundation, have recognized these changes in undergraduate medical education and have expressed serious concern regarding the marginalization of medical students, which has occurred in recent years.[6,7] The AAMC has launched the Project on the Clinical Education of Medical Students in an attempt to combat this trend, and the Carnegie Foundation has called for better standardization of outcomes across medical schools with a focus on tailoring learning needs to students' future residency and career choices.

ENTRUSTABLE PROFESSIONAL ACTIVITIES

In recognition of this variation in preparation across medical schools, the AAMC has outlined 13 entrustable professional activities (EPAs) expected of all medical graduates I the United States (**Box 1**).[8] The EPAs are defined as "tasks or responsibilities that trainees are entrusted to perform unsupervised once they have attained sufficient

---

Box 1
Entrustable professional activities expected of all medical school graduates, as defined by the American Association of Medical Colleges

1. Gather a history and perform a physical examination.

2. Prioritize a differential diagnosis after a clinical encounter.

3. Recommend and interpret common diagnostic and screening tests.

4. Enter and discuss orders and prescriptions.

5. Document a clinical encounter in the patient record.

6. Provide an oral presentation of a clinical encounter.

7. Form clinical questions and retrieve evidence to advance patient care.

8. Give or receive a patient handover to transition care responsibility.

9. Collaborate as a member of an interprofessional team.

10. Recognize a patient requiring urgent or emergent care and initiate evaluation and management.

11. Obtain informed consent for tests and/or procedures.

12. Perform general procedures of a physician.

13. Identify system failures and contribute to a culture of safety and improvement.

From AAMC. Core entrustable professional activities for entering residency. American Association of Medical Colleges. 2014; with permission.

---

specific competence."[8] Within each EPA are a number of areas of competency with associated milestones defined, and a learner progresses from "pre-entrustable" to "entrustable" levels based on their performance in each competency domain. The EPAs expected to be mastered by all medical students are foundational skills that all physicians should possess, such as "gather a history and perform a physical examination," "give or receive a patient handover to transition care responsibility," or "obtain informed consent for tests and/or procedures." Attainment of competence in these EPAs is not time based, however, and allows for additional specialty specific EPAs to be defined as well within the medical school curriculum. A number of specialties have defined specific EPAs tailored to their specialty training, and some of these EPAs are expected to be attained during medical school, as demonstrated by the approach taken by the pediatrics community.[9–11]

Surgery educators have an opportunity to use this concept of EPAs to define more explicitly the goals of residency training. Once outlined, EPAs can be implemented across both residency programs as well as within undergraduate medical education. In addition to achieving basic competency in the 13 core EPAs defined by the AAMC, medical students could similarly demonstrate competency in surgical EPAs, allowing them to better progress into residency training with defined competence in specific domains. This achievement would significantly ease the burden on program directors as they safely transition new PGY1 residents into residency with the appropriate level of supervision.

IMPACT ON CAREER CHOICE AND RETENTION IN GENERAL SURGERY

A perhaps underconsidered aspect of the ongoing concerns regarding the current limited exposure of medical students in the clinical environment is the potential impact on their career selection. A student who is underexposed to their specialty of choice during medical school may enter the field of surgery without a clear understanding of the nature and rigors of a surgery residency and future practice as a result. A surgery residency continues to be difficult, with some of the highest hours in postgraduate training; if students lack adequate understanding of the challenges that they will encounter, they may be more likely to suffer burnout and dissatisfaction.

General surgery residencies have long experienced a higher attrition rate than some other surgery fields, and educators have long sought to understand and to positively impact this phenomenon. Initially, it was hypothesized that the institution of the Accreditation Council for Graduate Medical Education duty-hour regulations would improve attrition rates by leveling the hours requirements compared with other specialties.[12] However, several studies found that the attrition rate has remained high and perhaps even increased since the 2003 duty-hour regulations.[13,14] It may be that the duty-hour regulations increased the appeal of general surgery residencies, giving applicants a false sense of security regarding the difficulty of a surgery residency. In a recent national study of attrition, the authors found that the attrition rate in general surgery remains at approximately 20% across all programs, and that attrition occurs most commonly in intern year; the authors suggest in their discussion that this may reflect students lacking adequate exposure to and understanding of the nature of a career in surgery.[15] Therefore, a potential avenue for improvement is to increase our efforts and involvement earlier in medical education, to ensure that students are making an adequately informed career choice before entering residency.

In addition, earlier and more comprehensive involvement in undergraduate medical education may enable surgery educators to more proactively identify and recruit students likely to succeed in a career in surgery. Along with the attention paid to attrition have come complementary efforts to identify the traits associated with success. The National Study of Expectations and Attitudes of Residents in Surgery survey has been used to profile resident attitudes and identify factors that put trainees at risk for attrition[16]; more recently a novel psychological profiling tool—grit—has been suggested for identifying those likely to succeed in residency.[17] Measuring grit and attitude are formidable tasks to undertake in a short meeting of an applicant during general residency interviews; however, educators who develop more substantial interactions and relationships with students earlier in their medical training may be able to better parse out these metrics over time and guide students toward career choices that optimally position them for success.

FOURTH YEAR PREPARATORY COURSES: SURGERY "BOOT CAMP"

Efforts to improve students' preparedness for surgical internship have largely been positioned in the fourth year of medical school. The rationale for this is primarily one of convenience and tradition, because students have selected their career path at this point and are therefore motivated to pursue further preparation in surgery, and medical schools have flexible fourth-year curricula that allow for tailored experiences. Over the past decades, a number of medical schools have developed intern preparatory electives, intended to provide practical training for students entering surgery residencies.[18–21] These electives often combine didactic teaching, simulation experiences, and technical skills training with suture laboratories, cadaver and animal dissection, and laparoscopic simulators.

The strength of these preparatory courses lies in their timing; the majority are scheduled in the spring of the fourth year, in close proximity to the start of residency training. This lends itself to skill and knowledge retention over the short term and students are typically well-motivated during this period because they are anxious about their own level of preparedness. A number of studies have demonstrated that these elective courses are effective in improving trainees' confidence and reducing anxiety. A recent metaanalysis summarized the findings of single-institution retrospective studies of intern preparatory courses, finding that there were significant improvements in the domains of technical skill, clinical knowledge, and self-confidence.[22]

What the existing literature lacks, however, is evidence of how this short-term boost in confidence translates into long-term performance in residency itself. Although intern preparatory courses have been underway at a few medical schools for more than a decade, the majority of these courses are in their nascence, and to date it has been difficult to track the performance of graduates of these boot camp courses once they matriculate into their residencies. Further, similar to the variation in other parts of medical schools' curricula, these boot camp courses have historically been varied in the depth and content provided.

MOVING TOWARD A COMMON PREPARATORY CURRICULUM: IDENTIFYING CORE ELEMENTS

Given the concerns for variation in medical school graduates' readiness for transitioning to their new roles as PGY1 residents, the American College of Surgeons (ACS), Association of Program Directors in Surgery (APDS), and Association for Surgical Education (ASE) have collaborated to not only promote these intern preparatory courses, but to enhance and standardize their content. These organizations have developed a joint task force to improve medical students' readiness for entering surgery, namely, the ACS/APDS/ASE Resident Prep Curriculum Committee.[23] At the outset of this joint initiative, a needs assessment was performed across multiple institutions to better understand the current gaps in training in medical school with respect to skills needed upon entry into surgery residency, and secondarily to assess the impact of an fourth year preparatory curriculum.[1]

To perform this mixed methods needs assessment, interns across multiple institutions were surveyed regarding their preparedness for their intern year, asked to describe their most challenging situation that had encountered in residency thus far, and asked to comment as to their level of preparedness to manage that situation. The interns surveyed responded that, in retrospect, they felt that their medical school training left them only "moderately" prepared to care for a variety of common postoperative conditions, such as managing hypotension or electrolyte abnormalities, as well as feeling unprepared for emergent bedside procedures. Interns also reported feeling only moderately comfortable prescribing common perioperative drugs such as antibiotics and antihypertensives, and felt only moderately comfortable writing patient care and admission orders. Interns expressed significant anxiety regarding efficiency and time management aspects of the PGY1 year, that is, triaging multiple simultaneous demands, as well as toward being first responders for unstable patients. In reviewing the responses of interns, a panel of surgery educators felt that the overwhelming majority of these challenging scenarios would be amenable to training and that these specific scenarios could be easily incorporated into an fourth year preparatory course.[1]

Using this needs assessment, the ACS/APDS/ASE task force identified a number of critical core elements of a preparatory curriculum that should be incorporated into all courses and that are anchored to the Accreditation Council for Graduate Medical Education PGY1 supervision requirements. Goals and objectives have been defined to support the ACS/APDS/ASE Resident Prep Curriculum, and modular content has been collected or developed that can be disseminated across medical schools to aid in course development.[23] Common modules used to meet the goals and objectives of the course are:

- A common call/mock paging program to cover common clinical scenarios encountered by interns.
- Simulated patient scenarios to give medical students practice being first responders to acute situations; hands-on order entry and prescribing practice.
- Technical skills training with focus on both operative skills, such as knot-tying and suturing, as well as simulated bedside procedures such as ultrasound-guided central line placement.
- Radiographic image interpretation practice.
- Operative anatomy experience, through animate or cadaveric laboratory sessions.

The response to the development of this multidimensional, flexible curriculum with standard goals and objectives has been met with great enthusiasm. Although only in its third year of offering, more than 45 medical schools are now participating with continued expressed interest from other medical schools. Other stakeholders in the surgery community have also recognized the value of this initiative and the approach of incorporating dedicated training into medical school for surgery residency, with a call for all incoming PGY1 residents to complete such a curriculum of blended learning.[24–29] It is important to emphasize the active nature of this curriculum, and further detail regarding some of the key modules offered is provided herein.

Mock Paging Programs

One of the most anxiety-provoking experiences for new interns is responding to floor pages on potentially ill patients. Very few students gain adequate exposure to this experience in their medical school clerkships owing to the previously outlined concerns for marginalization during their clinical rotations. Educators at Southern Illinois University have developed a robust program to provide students this experience through a series of standardized simulated patient scenarios.[30] Trained nurses page students with a detailed clinical scenario; when students call back, they are asked to gather information through the nurse and initiate an appropriate action plan. Each scenario has been developed by a team of surgeons and nurses, and students are given a standardized evaluation of their performance. In addition to the challenge of the clinical scenario, these simulated scenarios allow students to be confronted by communication challenges, such as an inexperienced nurse who cannot provide complete information regarding the patient's condition. The pages also come at unexpected hours, even late at night, to simulate the spontaneity and unpredictability of taking call. Immediately after the call, the student is called back and provided with feedback regarding their management of the case as well as their communication style.

This mock paging program has been well-studied; participants have improved their clinical performance significantly and participants of the program have expressed decreased anxiety and increased confidence regarding their ability to respond to clinical pages as a resident.[30]

Interactive Patient Care Scenarios

The online preparatory curriculum includes a series of modules for common clinical scenarios that take students through an interactive clinical case, including preoperative risk assessment and perioperative care.[23] These scenarios allow for student interaction and discussion as well as presentation of evidence-based guidelines. In addition, they allow for simulated order entry and discussion of perioperative care.

Technical Skills Training

The common preparatory curriculum includes a robust series of technical skills training exercises. Open operative techniques, including fundamental skills such as knot tying and suturing, are emphasized and assessed. In addition, simulation facilities can be used to incorporate bedside procedures, such as central line placement as well as laparoscopic task trainers. There is an existing body of evidence to support the usefulness and durability of early skills acquisition through simulation-based training programs such as these.[31–34]

VISION FOR THE FUTURE: INTEGRATING LONGITUDINAL EFFORTS THROUGHOUT MEDICAL SCHOOL

At present, many efforts have focused on improving preparation for a career in surgery through these late electives and experience during the fourth year of medical school. Moving forward, surgeon–educators need to proactively involve themselves earlier in medical school, both in the traditional third year clerkship as well as through efforts in the preclinical years. Surgery mentoring programs for first and second year medical students have received a great deal of attention; however, these efforts are often fragmented experiences and separate from the core learning activities of the M1 and M2 years.[35] The ACS and ASE have attempted to improve on these efforts by developing a simulation-based surgery skills curriculum for integration across the early years of medical school.[36] This curriculum has 25 online modules, with both content as well as assessment tools, covering a variety of early skills that can be taught before students entering their core surgical clerkships (**Box 2**). Through these efforts, the hope is that more integrated involvement in procedural training can be incorporated throughout medical school. Although the skills included in this curriculum are meant to be for all graduating physicians regardless of specialty, integration of this curriculum in the early years of medical school provides an opportunity for surgeons to interact with students from the beginning of medical school. Students would progress through core EPAs, basics of procedural skills, and then move into more advanced surgery-specific preparation through subinternships and preparatory courses (**Fig. 1**); in this way students would enter residency with a more consistent baseline set of skills and the variation seen between graduates at present should be reduced.

Although these online modules are promising, more transformative changes are needed to improve our current approach to undergraduate medical education. To that end, the American Medical Association has developed a large-scale initiative entitled "Accelerating Change in Medical Education"[37]; this project has endowed grants to 11 medical schools to radically redesign their approach to clinical education. At a number of these institutions, including our own, this change has come through a longitudinally integrated clinical curriculum that intertwines early clinical experiences with the traditional basic science foundation of medical education. These changes in education offer an opportunity for surgery educators to take part in this early integration of clinical experiences, and should improve students' exposure to career paths in surgery throughout medical school. At the University of Michigan, this curriculum redesign has been envisioned as a "trunk and branches" architecture, with the "trunk" consisting of the foundational knowledge needed for all medical practitioners, and the "branches" allowing students to embark on an intentional pathway of clinical learning tailored to their personal interests (**Fig. 2**).[38] In the initial stages of the

---

Box 2
ACS/ASE medical student simulation-based surgical skills curriculum

Year 1

1. Abdominal examination
2. Basic vascular examination
3. Breast examination
4. Digital rectal examination
5. Female pelvic examination
6. Male groin and genital examination
7. Universal precautions
8. Venipuncture

Year 2

1. Basic airway management
2. Communication: History and physical examination
3. Foley bladder catheterization
4. Intermediate vascular examination
5. Nasogastric tubes
6. Sterile technique: Gloving and gowning
7. Surgical drains: Care and removal

Year 3

1. Arterial puncture and blood gas
2. Basic knot tying
3. Basic suturing
4. Central venous line insertion
5. Communication: Codes, safe and effective handoffs
6. Intermediate airway
7. Intraosseous IV
8. Local anesthetics
9. Paracentesis
10. Thoracentesis

Adapted from ACS/ASE medical student simulation based surgical skills curriculum. American College of Surgeons 2014.

---

redesigned medical curriculum, there are 5 clinical and scientific branches: patients and populations, procedure-based care, diagnostic and therapeutic technologies, system and hospital focused practice, and blended/flexible. The procedure-based care branch offers a unique pathway for students interested in careers in surgery, and our hope is that this pathway will allow for early, deliberate, and consistent interaction between general surgery faculty and interested medical students. **Fig. 3** demonstrates a sample schedule for a particular type of student planning to pursue a career in surgery. Students with alternate goals or needs would have a modified schedule designed to maximize their success.

Year 1	Year 2	Year 3	Year 4
AAMC Medical Student Core EPAs			Surgery Specific EPAs
ACS/ASE M1-M3 Skills Curriculum			
		ACS/ASE M3 Curriculum	ACS/APDS/ASE Prep Curriculum
			ASE M4 Sub-I Curriculum

Fig. 1. Proposed longitudinal integration of surgery training throughout medical school. AAMC, Association of American Medical Colleges; ACS, American College of Surgeons; ASE, Association for Surgical Education; APDS, Association of Program Directors in Surgery; EPAs, Entrustable Professional Activities.

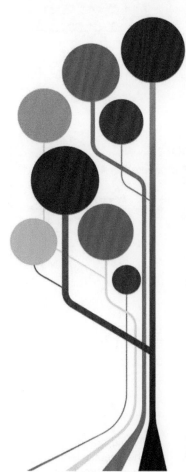

FOURTH YEAR / LATE BRANCHES

As students progress along the branches, they will gain greater clinical skills and professional self-understanding to make meaningful choices in their education on their path as physician leaders.

THIRD YEAR / EARLY BRANCHES

Students will develop an advanced professional identity and commitment to a chosen professional focus. The early Branches will give students the opportunity to explore the different areas of medicine within a supportive structure.

SECOND YEAR / CLINICAL TRUNK

Students will learn the foundations of patient care. The Clinical Trunk features two phases of learning in the clinical environment. In the first phase, students will evaluate patients with core conditions and receive observation and feedback on clinical skills. In the second phase students will be immersed in departmentally administered clinical care teams.

FIRST YEAR / SCIENTIFIC TRUNK

To give students an integrated understanding of the foundational medical sciences. The Scientific Trunk features organ-system-based sequences, a "chief complaint" curriculum to develop clinical reasoning skills, and an "optimizing patient care curriculum" to develop skills and habits of information management.

INTEGRATED LEARNING Throughout each year of your educational experience, there will be meaningful clinical learning, application of relevance science, leadership development training, and a learning community to foster professional growth.

Fig. 2. University of Michigan curriculum trunk and branches model flow diagram. (*Adapted from* University of Michigan Medical School. Branches: advanced professional development. Available at: http://curriculum.med.umich.edu; with permission. Available at: http://curriculum.med.umich.edu/curriculum/branches; Accessed September 15, 2015.)

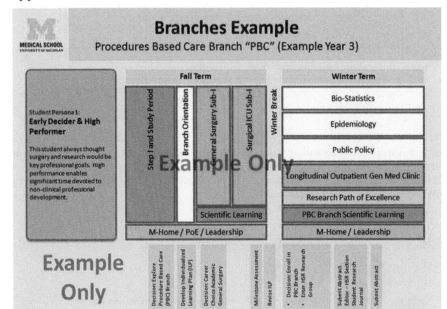

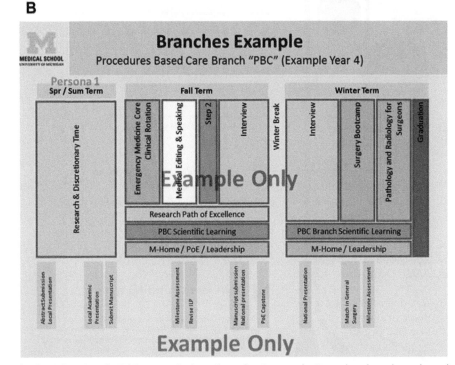

Fig. 3. University of Michigan curriculum "branches" example: Procedure based care branch years 3 (A) and 4 (B) curricula for a single potential student type (persona 1). Experiences would be modified for students with alternate goals or needs. Gen Med, general medicine; PoE, path of excellence; Spr, spring; Sum, summer. (*Adapted from* University of Michigan Medical School. Branches: advanced professional development. Available at: http://curriculum.med.umich.edu; with permission. Available at: http://curriculum.med.umich.edu/curriculum/branches; Accessed September 15, 2015.)

Similar models for allowing early differentiation and tailoring of educational experience are in development at a variety of medical schools. The New York University School of Medicine has taken the idea of even further, allowing students to apply to an accelerated 3-year medical school curriculum with a joint acceptance into residency programs in their chosen field of interest upon completion of medical schools.[39] Twenty different residency programs at the New York University Langone Medical Center are participating in this initiative, including general surgery. Our hope is that, moving forward, these various pilot initiatives will help us to plot a course to integrate surgery training throughout undergraduate medical education, improving the preparedness of graduates and enabling better understanding on their part of what a career in surgery entails. This experience should in turn better serve the patients that these graduates will care for as they move into surgery residency and on into their careers in surgery.

SUMMARY

The ACS, APDS, and ASE have made strides toward longitudinal integration in medical education; however, the bulk of ongoing efforts have focused on the fourth year of training, because medical students have declared their interest in surgery and are relatively differentiated at this point. Although these current efforts to improve preparation are promising, surgery educators need to further invest in medical student training across all years of medical school if we are to make a substantial impact and help improve readiness for graduates to embark on a career in surgery.

REFERENCES

1. Minter RM, Amos KD, Bentz ML, et al. Transition to surgical residency: a multi-institutional study of perceived intern preparedness and the effect of a formal residency preparatory course in the fourth year of medical school. Acad Med 2015; 90(8):1116–24.
2. Sachdeva AK, Loiacono LA, Amiel GE, et al. Variability in the clinical skills of residents entering training programs in surgery. Surgery 1995;118:300–8 [discussion: 308–9].
3. Lyss-Lerman P, Teherani A, Aagaard E, et al. What training is needed in the fourth year of medical school? Views of residency program directors. Acad Med 2009; 84:823–9.
4. Walling A, Merando A. The fourth year of medical education: a literature review. Acad Med 2010;85:1698–704.
5. AAMC Compliance Advisory. Electronic health records in academic health centers. 2011.
6. American Association of Medical Colleges Project on the clinical education of medical students. 2010.
7. Irby DM, Cooke M, O'Brien BC. Calls for reform of medical education by the Carnegie Foundation for the Advancement of Teaching: 1910 and 2010. Acad Med 2010;85:220–7.
8. AAMC. Core entrustable professional activities for entering residency. American Association of Medical Colleges; 2014.
9. Hauer KE, Kohlwes J, Cornett P, et al. Identifying entrustable professional activities in internal medicine training. J Grad Med Educ 2013;5:54–9.
10. Caverzagie KJ, Cooney TG, Hemmer PA, et al. The development of entrustable professional activities for internal medicine residency training: a report from the

Education Redesign Committee of the Alliance for Academic Internal Medicine. Acad Med 2015;90:479–84.

11. Shaughnessy AF, Sparks J, Cohen-Osher M, et al. Entrustable professional activities in family medicine. J Grad Med Educ 2013;5:112–8.

12. Arnold MW, Patterson AF, Tang AS. Has implementation of the 80-hour work week made a career in surgery more appealing to medical students? Am J Surg 2005; 189:129–33.

13. Everett CB, Helmer SD, Osland JS, et al. General surgery resident attrition and the 80-hour workweek. Am J Surg 2007;194:751–6 [discussion: 756–7].

14. Naylor RA, Reisch JS, Valentine RJ. Factors related to attrition in surgery residency based on application data. Arch Surg 2008;143:647–51 [discussion: 651–2].

15. Yeo H, Bucholz E, Ann Sosa J, et al. A national study of attrition in general surgery training: which residents leave and where do they go? Ann Surg 2010;252: 529–34 [discussion: 534–6].

16. Yeo H, Viola K, Berg D, et al. Attitudes, training experiences, and professional expectations of US general surgery residents: a national survey. JAMA 2009; 302:1301–8.

17. Burkhart RA, Tholey RM, Guinto D, et al. Grit: a marker of residents at risk for attrition? Surgery 2014;155:1014–22.

18. Boehler ML, Rogers DA, Schwind CJ, et al. A senior elective designed to prepare medical students for surgical residency. Am J Surg 2004;187:695–7.

19. Esterl RM Jr, Henzi DL, Cohn SM. Senior medical student "boot camp": can result in increased self-confidence before starting surgery internships. Curr Surg 2006; 63:264–8.

20. Meier AH, Henry J, Marine R, et al. Implementation of a Web- and simulation-based curriculum to ease the transition from medical school to surgical internship. Am J Surg 2005;190:137–40.

21. Teo AR, Harleman E, O'Sullivan PS, et al. The key role of a transition course in preparing medical students for internship. Acad Med 2011;86:860–5.

22. Blackmore C, Austin J, Lopushinsky SR, et al. Effects of postgraduate medical education "boot camps" on clinical skills, knowledge, and confidence: a meta-analysis. J Grad Med Educ 2014;6:643–52.

23. ACS/APDS/ASE Resident Prep Curriculum. 2015.

24. American Board of Surgery, American College of Surgeons, Association of Program Directors in Surgery, Association for Surgical Education. Statement on surgical preresidency preparatory courses. Surgery 2014;156:1059–60.

25. American Board of Surgery, American College of Surgeons, Association of Program Directors in Surgery, Association for Surgical Education. Statement on surgical pre-residency preparatory courses. JAMA Surg 2014;149:1198–9.

26. American Board of Surgery, American College of Surgeons, Association of Program Directors in Surgery, Association for Surgical Education. Statement on surgical preresidency preparatory courses. Am J Surg 2014;208:695–6.

27. American Board of Surgery, American College of Surgeons, Association of Program Directors in Surgery, Association for Surgical Education. Statement on surgical pre-residency preparatory courses. World J Surg 2014;38:2743–5.

28. American Board of Surgery, American College of Surgeons, Association of Program Directors in Surgery, Association for Surgical Education. Statement on surgical pre-residency preparatory courses. J Am Coll Surg 2014;219:851–2.

29. Association of Program Directors in Surgery, American Board of Surgery, American College of Surgeons, Association for Surgical Education. Statement on surgical preresidency preparatory courses. Ann Surg 2014;260:969–70.

30. Frischknecht AC, Boehler ML, Schwind CJ, et al. How prepared are your interns to take calls? Results of a multi-institutional study of simulated pages to prepare medical students for surgery internship. Am J Surg 2014;208:307–15.
31. Sturm LP, Windsor JA, Cosman PH, et al. A systematic review of skills transfer after surgical simulation training. Ann Surg 2008;248:166–79.
32. Sutherland LM, Middleton PF, Anthony A, et al. Surgical simulation: a systematic review. Ann Surg 2006;243:291–300.
33. Tavakol M, Mohagheghi MA, Dennick R. Assessing the skills of surgical residents using simulation. J Surg Educ 2008;65:77–83.
34. Thomas RE, Crutcher R, Lorenzetti D. A systematic review of the methodological quality and outcomes of RCTs to teach medical undergraduates surgical and emergency procedures. Can J Surg 2007;50:278–90.
35. Sammann A, Tendick F, Ward D, et al. A surgical skills elective to expose preclinical medical students to surgery. J Surg Res 2007;142:287–94.
36. ACS/ASE medical student simulation based surgical skills curriculum. American College of Surgeons; 2014.
37. American Medical Association. Accelerating change in medical education. 2014.
38. University of Michigan Medical School. Curriculum strategic planning. 2015.
39. NYU School of Medicine. Three-year MD pathway. 2014.

Assessment of Competence
The Accreditation Council for Graduate Medical Education/Residency Review Committee Perspective

John R. Potts III, MD[a,b,c],*

KEYWORDS

- Competencies • Outcomes project • Milestones
- Clinical Learning Environment Review • Competency-based resident education

KEY POINTS

- Competence is an individual trait that is task-specific and inconstant.
- The ACGME does not define or evaluate individual competence but has, in the past 15 years, promulgated several initiatives to help programs assess competence in their residents and fellows.
- In the near future, the ACGME will implement an initiative by which programs can develop and study the results of competency-based residency curricula.

THE ACCREDITATION COUNCIL FOR GRADUATE MEDICAL EDUCATION COMPETENCIES

What are frequently referred to as the Accreditation Council for Graduate Medical Education (ACGME) competencies were actually the product of a combined effort by the ACGME and the American Board of Medical Specialties (ABMS). That work began in earnest in 1999 and, for the ACGME, was central to the rollout of The Outcomes Project in 2000 to 2001. The brief descriptors of those six competencies are discussed next.[1]

Patient Care

Residents must be able to provide patient care that is compassionate, appropriate, and effective for the treatment of health problems and the promotion of health.

Disclosures: The author is a full-time employee of the Accreditation Council for Graduate Medical Education and has no other relevant disclosures.
[a] ACGME, 515 N. State Street, Suite 2000, Chicago, IL 60654, USA; [b] Department of Surgery, University of Texas Houston Medical School, 6431 Fannin Street, Houston, TX 77030, USA; [c] Department of Medical Education, University of Illinois at Chicago College of Medicine, 808 S. Wood Street, M/C 591, Chicago, IL 60612, USA
* ACGME, 515 N. State Street, Suite 2000, Chicago, IL 60654.
E-mail address: jpotts@acgme.org

Residents must be able to competently perform all medical, diagnostic, and surgical procedures considered essential for the area of practice.

Medical Knowledge

Residents must demonstrate knowledge of established and evolving biomedical, clinical, epidemiologic, and social-behavioral sciences, and the application of this knowledge to patient care.

Practice-Based Learning and Improvement

Residents must demonstrate the ability to investigate and evaluate their care of patients, to appraise and assimilate scientific evidence, and to continuously improve patient care based on constant self-evaluation and life-long learning. Residents are expected to develop skills and habits to be able to meet the following goals: identify strengths, deficiencies, and limits in one's knowledge and expertise; set learning and improvement goals; identify and perform appropriate learning activities; systematically analyze practice using quality improvement methods, and implement changes with the goal of practice improvement and incorporate formative evaluation feedback into daily practice; locate, appraise, and assimilate evidence from scientific studies related to their patients' health problems; use information technology to optimize learning; and participate in the education of patients, families, students, residents, and other health professionals.

Interpersonal and Communication Skills

Residents must demonstrate interpersonal and communication skills that result in the effective exchange of information and collaboration with patients, their families, and health professionals. Residents are expected to communicate effectively with patients, families, and the public, as appropriate, across a broad range of socioeconomic and cultural backgrounds; communicate effectively with physicians, other health professionals, and health-related agencies; work effectively as a member or leader of a health care team or other professional group; act in a consultative role to other physicians and health professionals; and maintain comprehensive, timely, and legible medical records, if applicable.

Professionalism

Residents must demonstrate a commitment to carrying out professional responsibilities and an adherence to ethical principles. Residents are expected to demonstrate compassion, integrity, and respect for others; responsiveness to patient needs that supersedes self-interest; respect for patient privacy and autonomy; accountability to patients, society, and the profession; and sensitivity and responsiveness to a diverse patient population, including but not limited to diversity in gender, age, culture, race, religion, disabilities, and sexual orientation.

Systems-Based Practice

Residents must demonstrate an awareness of and responsiveness to the larger context and system of health care, and the ability to call effectively on other resources in the system to provide optimal health care. Residents are expected to work effectively in various health care delivery settings and systems relevant to their clinical specialty, coordinate patient care within the health care system relevant to their clinical specialty, incorporate considerations of cost awareness and risk-benefit analysis in patient and/or population-based care as appropriate, advocate for quality patient care and optimal patient care systems, work in interprofessional teams to enhance patient safety and improve patient care quality, and participate in identifying system errors and implementing potential systems solutions.

Limitations

Although they were an important step forward in the assessment of competence in GME, multiple limitations have been recognized with the competencies. Although patient care, medical knowledge, interpersonal and communications skills, and professionalism were intuitively understood by educators and learners, the concepts of practice-based learning and improvement and systems-based practice were not. A substantial amount of effort has been expended educating the educators at the national and local level regarding those two competencies, first as to what they are and then in ways to teach and assess them.

Other limitations of the competencies have been noted by Ginsberg and coworkers.[2] In the clinical workplace arena, the six competencies are overlapping and interdependent and cannot be independently assessed. Competence develops through experience, is not a stable trait, and is inherently subjective. Furthermore, the expertise of raters (as clinicians and as raters) is variable and, itself, not stable. Finally, Ginsberg and coworkers[2] point out that the social encounter context of the clinical workplace contributes to uneven assessment of competence.

Although the ACGME Common and Specialty Program Requirements frequently invoke the words competence, competent, and competently, they do not define clinical competence. One reason that the ACGME requirements do not define clinical competence is that clinical competence is an individual trait and the ACGME does not certify individuals. As an accreditor, the focus of ACGME is on the ability of a program and institution to provide the educational environment and resources necessary to train competent physicians and surgeons. Operative case requirements stand as an exemplar. The ACGME Review Committee for Surgery has for decades had minimum case requirements in multiple categories. The program requirements for GME in general surgery clearly state, however, that, "Performance of this minimum number of cases by a resident must not be interpreted as an equivalent to competence achievement."[3] The review committee has established minima to ensure that an accredited program can provide a sufficient breadth and depth of operative experience for the training of surgeons.

COMPETENCE

Competence is somewhat ill-defined. One dictionary defines "competent" as an adjective meaning, "Having the necessary ability, knowledge, or skill to do something successfully"[4] (interestingly, the example provided with that definition is "a highly competent surgeon"). Nevertheless, competence is usually easily recognized when it is observed and even more easily recognized in its absence. One might be a competent surgeon with high levels of attainment of the six competencies discussed previously, but one could not be a competent surgeon absent high levels of attainment of those six competencies. This is certainly true of the technical skill aspect of patient care because it is technical ability that distinguishes surgeons from all other medical practitioners. Competency is a task-specific trait, whether that task be technical or otherwise. It is imperative to recognize and remember that (as noted by Ginsberg and coworkers[2]) competency is not a stable condition. Although one may have demonstrably achieved competency in a given task today, that same individual may or may not be able to demonstrate competency in the same task tomorrow or a year from now or a decade from now. In some part (particularly for such physical achievements as technical skill) this is a result of the physiologic limitations and consequences of aging. However, on a day-to-day basis, it can be the manifestation of the degree of intentional practice of the task. Numerous other forces can disrupt that fleeting state of competence including (but not limited to) fatigue and other forms of impairment. In summary, competency is an ill-defined but observable task-specific and unstable condition of individuals.

The ACGME does not and cannot assess competence. As an accrediting agency, the ACGME can and does attempt to improve the ability of GME programs to produce competent physicians and surgeons through changes in standards, education, and assessment of programs and institutions.

THE EDUCATIONAL ENVIRONMENT
Federal Regulation

The educational environment of GME programs has been altered dramatically over the past three decades. In no small part, this has been due to regulations associated with the substantial contribution of federal funding to GME. The "cap" on GME training slots has forced institutions to make difficult financial, administrative, and clinical decisions to regulate the growth of GME programs and positions. The regulations regarding Medicare payments to teaching faculty in GME programs (and the consequences of failing to strictly adhere to those regulations) has unintentionally had a major and negative impact on the appropriate supervision of residents in the designed transition to independent practice. The electronic medical record, which is often thought of more as a billing tool than a tool for patient care, now consumes substantial portions of residents' days. The consolidation of health care into fewer and fewer and larger and larger corporations undoubtedly also impacts (in ways yet to be fully understood) the environment of GME.

The Accreditation Council for Graduate Medical Education Outcomes Project

For its part, perhaps the first major perturbation of the educational environment by the ACGME was the introduction of the competencies in the Outcomes Project, which was originally initiated in 1997.[5] That initiative marked the first time that resident educators were systematically asked to dissect what they taught and assessed into component parts. That the ACGME could define the six competencies in terms common to all specialties in the Common Program Requirements codified the similarities across the practice of medicine, regardless of specialty. The specialty-specific requirements added by each review committee emphasized and codified the specialty differences.

Milestones

Building on the Outcomes Project and the competencies, the Milestones project was initiated in about 2009.[6] The Milestones are an initiative of the ACGME but deliberately and consistently involved the ABMS member boards, program director groups, specialty academies and colleges and residents to represent the breadth across each specialty. The general idea of the Milestones is to formulate more explicit definitions of the knowledge, skills, attributes, and performance expected of residents and fellows using the competency framework and to identify and delineate the time course commonly experienced by those trainees in achieving them. As such, the Milestones serve as a roadmap for the individual developing through residency and fellowship. They can also serve as a tool for assessment of competency during that development. Importantly, that assessment does not depend on a written examination of knowledge or an oral examination of what the trainee says she or he would do or a simulated experience. The assessment of Milestones occurs in the clinical workplace and is, therefore, reflective of what residents actually do.

Because the Milestones are assessed using multiple evaluations from multiple evaluators in multiple settings, they are reflective of the level of performance of the trainee day-in and day-out. The assessment of the Milestones is not only of importance to the individual trainee and to the individual GME program. It is important to GME (writ large) because when used collectively the Milestones provide the best opportunity yet to demonstrate to the public that funds GME that learning actually occurs in GME programs. To be feasible, the Milestones represent only a small sample of all of the knowledge, skills, attributes, and performance expected of trainees and simply cannot exhaustively represent the entire spectrum of what a trainee is to learn and demonstrate. Nevertheless, they stand as an important contribution to the learning and the assessment of that learning in GME programs.

The Next Accreditation System

In 2006, the ACGME developed a strategic plan with four major components[7]: (1) foster innovation and improvement in the learning environment, (2) increase the accreditation emphasis on educational outcomes, (3) increase efficiency and reduce the burden of accreditation, and (4) improve the communication and collaboration with key internal and external stakeholders.

As a result of that strategic plan, the Next Accreditation System (NAS) was conceived and designed in 2012.[8] The NAS uses annually reported data rather than frequent site visits as the basis for accreditation decisions for programs and institutions. In-depth site visits are the only way that some information can be collected and are the only way that program-reported information can be systematically validated. Thus, even in the NAS site visits to programs and institutions continue to occur. However, the frequency of site visits has been reduced to every 10 years unless evaluation of the annual data prompts a review committee to request one earlier for a specific program. This key structural component of the NAS, which was one way that the ACGME aimed to reduce the burden of accreditation on programs and institutions, stood in sharp contrast to the 2009 report of the Institute of Medicine, which called for annual site visits for every program.[9] Partially in response to that appeal from the Institute of Medicine but, more importantly, because of the recognition that GME programs occur in the setting of a clinical and educational environment that strongly influences the behaviors of learners and educators and is often largely beyond the control of any single program, the ACGME launched the Clinical Learning Environment Review (CLER) program in 2012 as the foundation of the NAS.[10]

The Clinical Learning Environment Review

The CLER, aimed at the institutional rather than the program level, has six focus areas: (1) patient safety, (2) resident/fellow supervision, (3) health care quality (including health care disparities), (4) transitions of care, (5) duty hours and fatigue management, and (6) professionalism. Each of those six areas had long existed in the ACGME Common Program Requirements but had not previously been subject to systematic scrutiny. In the CLER visit, those areas are each evaluated in light of the resources devoted to them by the institution; their understanding, performance, teaching, and evaluation by the faculty; their understanding and performance by the residents and fellows; how the institution measures its current standing in each of the six areas; and improvements in the six areas documented by the institution. CLER visits are due to occur at each institution every 18 to 24 months. All ACGME-accredited institutions consisting of three or more programs have now undergone at least one CLER visit. The sometimes unique structure and the number of smaller (one- to two-program) institutions necessitated variations on the protocol used in larger institutions and a ramp up of the number of trained CLER site visitors. Those factors delayed the onset of CLER visits to the smaller institutions but those are now also underway. The CLER program is, by ACGME policy,[11] not used in the accreditation of institutions or programs with the sole exception that failure of an institution to undergo a CLER visit can result in an adverse accreditation action for that institution and, as a result, against the accredited programs within that institution. Competency is an individual trait. The CLER program does not evaluate the competence of individual trainees or of the faculty members within an institution. However, the clinical and educational environment does influence the teaching and learning of the competencies and the development of competent physicians,[12] so it is anticipated that the CLER program will positively influence the competency of those trainees and faculty members, alike.

COMPETENCY-BASED RESIDENCY EDUCATION

The concept of competency-based residency education is simple: residents graduate from a program and are extended the privilege of unsupervised clinical practice once they have demonstrated sufficient competence in the necessary elements of the specialty rather than based on having completed a prescribed length of time in the residency program. In some ways, competency-based residency education is "back to the future." The first surgical residency program was not time based. Residents under Dr Halsted at Johns Hopkins were essentially apprentices. He knew each of them and their abilities very well based on personal observation. Those individuals completed the residency when Dr Halsted considered them capable of independent practice. But, as simple as it may be in concept, competency-based surgical education is challenging to implement.

Regulatory Obstacles

The regulatory obstacles to competency-based medical education originate in the federal government, the certifying boards, and the ACGME. Institutions and programs largely depend on Medicare funding of GME. The formulas that dictate the funding provided to those entities on an annual basis are curious creatures that some may find interesting but that are beyond the scope of this article. What is important to the topic at hand is that GME funding by Medicare is predicated on a time-based residency model. If the first GME program that an individual enters is a 3-year program (eg, internal medicine), that individual is fully funded by Medicare for only 3 years of GME, regardless of whether that individual should transfer to a 4-year program in emergency medicine, a 5-year program in general surgery, or a 7-year program in neurosurgery. By the same token, should an individual in a 5-year general surgery residency program require a period of remediation such that her or his residency extended beyond 5 years, that period beyond the 5 year mark is not fully funded by Medicare. The current Medicare funding system works well for the program and institution with a competency-based residency program in general surgery when an individual completes the course in 4, 4.5, or 5 years. It does not work well for the same program and institution when an individual takes 5.5 or 6 years to complete the course. The certifying boards also stand as an obstacle because they routinely specify the number of years in an accredited training program necessary to enter candidacy for certification. Similarly, the obstacle to competency-based residency education posed by the ACGME is that, in every specialty and subspecialty, the ACGME program requirements for specialty education state as a core requirement the length of time in years that a program must last. As discussed next, the ACGME has taken the first small step to remove that barrier.

Competency-Based Curricula

Although not easy to do so, it is conceivable that a specialty broadly represented by the ACGME review committee, the certifying board, the specialty academy or college, other specialty experts, and residents could generate a thorough, competency-based curriculum for national implementation, as they did with the Milestones. The Milestones in many specialties (including general surgery) came to fruition only after a great deal of time and effort was devoted by many individuals who overcame several false starts. The development of a national competency-based curriculum is much more daunting. However, more daunting than the creation of a competency-based resident curriculum is the implementation of such a curriculum at the local level.

Local Barriers

At the local level, implementation of a competency-based resident education system for most programs would require a great deal of faculty educational development in the principles of teaching, feedback, and evaluation. That faculty development effort would necessarily involve the faculty at every hospital or other clinical site used by the program. Only those faculty members and clinical sites willing to earnestly engage in those educational activities to a much greater extent than is found in most programs today could successfully engage in a competency-based residency curriculum. Such a curriculum would entail evaluation systems very different than those aimed at summative evaluations, as found in most programs today. Such a learner-focused curriculum would demand day-to-day and even moment-to-moment evaluation of every individual resident to determine in what areas she or he can and does demonstrate competence and in what areas she or he can advance and the pace at which that advancement can take place. The truly interactive involvement between the resident and the faculty member, between the faculty member and her or his colleagues, between the faculty members and the program director, and between the program director and the resident would have to reach and sustain levels rarely encountered in most programs today. Presumably, such a level of engagement in educational activities would result in at least some decrement in the clinical activity of those faculty members, which in most programs would result in a decrease in their clinical income. Most programs currently have no mechanism in place to compensate for such a decrease in the clinical income of the teaching faculty. Furthermore, a competency-based resident curriculum would almost certainly (at least from time to time) disrupt the resident rotation schedule, which would result in some services having a normal or greater than normal number of residents present, whereas others had fewer than normal or no residents present for a period of time.

A competency-based curriculum would demand that residents be given opportunities each day to perform at their highest level of competence. In doing so, the residents' performance would certainly at times spill over into levels at which they were not competent. Thus, a competency-based residency curriculum would require a willingness on the part of faculty members to allow residents to progress through an operation or any other form of clinical encounter to the point of their incompetence and confidence on the part of the faculty member in her or his own ability to do whatever necessary to "rescue" the patient when that point of resident incompetence is reached. In short, most programs would have to undergo great structural and cultural change to successfully implement a competency-based resident education system.

Accreditation Council for Graduate Medical Education Facilitation of Competency-Based Residency Education

No program could implement such a system overnight but at least one program in Canada has successfully implemented a competency-based resident education system with some degree of success.[13] There are at least a few programs in the United States that wish to do so, but because of core requirements by the ACGME, no program can currently do so. However, recognizing the potential for competency-based resident education, the ACGME has begun to develop a mechanism for programs to be given waivers from the requirements for the number of years of training and, perhaps, other core requirements that stand as obstacles to the implementation of competency-based training programs. At this writing, the details of that mechanism are not yet fully delineated but the principles are being formulated. In general, the process would include the following elements.

Implementation of a competency-based curriculum would lead to great perturbation within a residency program. For that reason, proposals for such curricula would be viewed by the ACGME as pilot research studies of a specified duration. A program (or group of programs) would be required to make application to the ACGME for waiver of the core requirement regarding program length (and any other necessary core requirements). Only applications from programs with the status of Continued Accreditation would be considered. The application would have to explain in detail the current structure of the program, the proposed structure of the program in terms of resident assignments ("rotations"), and the rationale for the new structure. It would also have to describe in detail proposed changes in the resident evaluation system and the faculty educational development that is planned for implementation of those changes. The program would be asked to fully delineate the resources (financial and otherwise) necessary to support the proposed restructuring. The program would have to provide evidence of support from the local GME committee and from the executive leadership of the hospitals and other clinical sites that would be affected by the proposed changes. The program would also have to provide evidence from the specialty certifying board that individuals who complete the proposed program would be admissible to the certification process. A clear description of the outcome measures that would be used to assess the success of the program would be required, including the plan for following the progress of the residents after completion of the program. The program would also have to provide a detailed plan for remediation of those residents who fail to satisfactorily progress through the curriculum.

A panel of education experts convened by the ACGME would review the study proposal to ensure that all of the appropriate educational aspects had been addressed. That panel could accept the proposal, reject it, or request revisions. Once the panel accepted the educational aspects of the proposal, the proposal would then advance to the ACGME specialty review committee. The review committee could then accept the proposal, reject it, or request revisions. Only when accepted by the expert panel and the review committee could the program invoke the proposed curricular modifications. The program would then be closely monitored by the expert educational panel and the specialty review committee throughout the period of the study. Such monitoring would include frequent progress reports from the program detailing what was working well, what was not working as planned, and any deviations from the original study proposal made by the program. Although it would be gratifying to see that a single program could successfully invoke a competency-based curriculum, the ACGME is necessarily interested in knowing the scalability and general applicability of such programs. For that reason, it is anticipated that multi-institution study proposals would be more favorably viewed than those from single programs. Again, it must be emphasized that at this writing the ACGME has approved only in concept the idea of accepting applications for competency-based residency curricular. The elements listed previously will probably be included but the details of the application, approval, and monitoring processes are yet to be fully delineated.

SUMMARY

Competence is an individual trait. Because the ACGME (through its review committees) is an accrediting organization dealing with programs and institutions and is not a certifying organization dealing with individuals, it does not define competence, nor does it assess competence. Nevertheless, several major initiatives of the ACGME in the past 15 years have targeted improved assessment of the competence of residents and fellows at the program level. Those initiatives include the Outcomes Project and the competencies that emerged as key elements of that project; the Milestones; and the CLER, which is the foundation for the NAS. In the near future, the ACGME will implement an initiative by which programs can develop and study the results of competency-based residency curricula.

REFERENCES

1. ACGME Common Program Requirements. Available at: http://www.acgme.org/acgmeweb/Portals/0/PFAssets/ProgramRequirements/CPRs_07012015.pdf. Accessed June 12, 2015.
2. Ginsburg S, McIlroy J, Oulanova O, et al. Toward authentic clinical evaluation: pitfalls in the pursuit of competency. Acad Med 2010;85(5):780–6.
3. ACGME Program Requirements for Graduate Medical Education in General Surgery. Available at: http://www.acgme.org/acgmeweb/Portals/0/PFAssets/ProgramRequirements/440_general_surgery_07012015.pdf. Accessed June 12, 2015.
4. Competent defined. Available at: http://www.oxforddictionaries.com/us/definition/american_english/. Accessed July 3, 2015.
5. Swing SR. The ACGME outcome project: retrospective and prospective. Med Teach 2007;29(7):648–54.
6. Sullivan G, Simpson D, Cooney T, et al. A milestone in the milestones movement: the JGME milestones supplement. J Grad Med Educ 2013;5(1):1–4.
7. Accreditation Council for Graduate Medical Education 2005-2006 Annual Report. Available at: https://www.acgme.org/acgmeweb/Portals/0/PDFs/an_2005-06AnnRep.pdf. Accessed June 14, 2015.
8. Nasca TJ, Philibert I, Brigham T, et al. The next GME accreditation system: rationale and benefits. N Engl J Med 2012;366:1051–6.
9. Ulmer C, Wolman DM, Johns MME, editors. Resident duty hours: enhancing sleep, supervision, and safety. Washington, DC: The National Academies Press; 2009.
10. Weiss KB, Wagner R, Nasca TJ. Development, testing, and implementation of the ACGME Clinical Learning Environment Review (CLER) program. J Grad Med Educ 2012;4(3):396–8.

11. Accreditation Council for Graduate Medical Education Policies and Procedures Effective: June 13, 2015. Available at: http://acgme.org/acgmeweb/Portals/0/PDFs/ab_ACGMEPoliciesProcedures.pdf. Accessed August 10, 2015.
12. Asch DA, Nicholson S, Srinivas S, et al. Evaluating obstetrical residency programs using patient outcomes. JAMA 2009;302(12):1277–83.
13. Ferguson PC, Kraemer W, Nousiainen M, et al. Three-year experience with an innovative, modular competency-based curriculum for orthopedic training. J Bone Joint Surg Am 2013;95(21):e166.

Transition from Training to Surgical Practice

Thomas H. Cogbill, MD*, Stephen B. Shapiro, MD

KEYWORDS

- Surgical education • Transition to practice programs • General surgery careers
- Onboarding programs • Mentoring

KEY POINTS

- A subset of current surgery residency graduates does not feel confident or optimally prepared to enter directly into general surgery practice. Solutions to this vexing problem include redesign of the residency curriculum, credentialing during residency to encourage graded responsibility, effective onboarding programs for new surgeons, and development of transition to practice (TTP) programs in general surgery.
- Onboarding programs for new surgeons in larger health systems should include formal mentoring, career counseling, and operative case proctoring by senior surgeons as well as objective review of surgical outcomes.
- Onboarding programs for new surgeons in isolated practices may rely on former teaching faculty members, unaffiliated regional surgeons, or distance learning techniques to provide mentoring, proctoring, and case reviews.
- TTP programs have been developed in general surgery to provide a 1-year postresidency experience with independent decision making, operative procedure autonomy, personal mentoring by senior surgeons, practice management skill acquisition, and periodic review of performance and surgical case outcomes.

INTRODUCTION

The transformation of a surgeon from chief surgical resident or subspecialty fellow to attending does not take place in a single day nor does it occur without considerable effort on the part of the new surgeon or interested colleagues. For this transformation to successfully occur while ensuring patient safety requires far more of a planned program of TTP than a simple sink or swim model. The recent trainee is quickly thrown into the care of numerous patients for whom the clinical decisions more often involve

There are no conflicts of interest to disclose.
Department of General and Vascular Surgery, Gundersen Health System, 1900 South Avenue C05-001, La Crosse, WI 54601, USA
* Corresponding author.
E-mail address: thcogbil@gundersenhealth.org

shades of gray rather than the black or white learned in residency. Nights on call bring patients with emergent surgical needs that require crisp decision making, leadership, and judgment, which rely on experience they may not yet possess. A new graduate may be asked to perform complex or unfamiliar operative cases for the first time without a teaching faculty member across the table. In addition to these clinical challenges, the new graduate must quickly master the many facets of the business side of surgery, including billing and coding, insurance contracts and authorization, purchasing of expensive medical equipment, and management of health care personnel. All of this often takes place in a completely unfamiliar institution with many colleagues who are both strangers and competitors and a novel electronic medical record. Variation in the preparation provided by different training programs as well as individual surgeon skill sets make this transition from trainee to staff surgeon unpredictable. For patients to be well served, a new surgeon to get off on the right foot and to be successful, and the surgical department that they join to be stable, this critical period in a young surgeon's career must be well orchestrated.

This article focuses on surgical residency graduates' preparedness for practice, important issues that currently revolve around the transition from training to practice, institutional methods of onboarding for new surgeons, the American College of Surgeons (ACS) TTP program, and future methods that might be used to assist in this transformational period.

ARE CURRENT RESIDENCY GRADUATES READY FOR SURGICAL PRACTICE?

Several recent trends concerning surgical education have resulted in significant challenges in the preparedness of current graduates.[1] Residency has de facto been shortened by nearly 12 months due to duty-hour restrictions. Although the total number of operative cases has remained stable, the number of emergency cases has diminished. Opportunities for autonomy and independent decision making during residency have become a rarity due to regulatory changes, medical-legal concerns, societal and ethical changes, and health care financing enforcement. The majority of surgical experience in most programs occurs on subspecialty surgical rotations and exposure to general surgeons is limited. Approximately 80% of graduates choose to pursue fellowship immediately after residency, leaving only 20% who enter surgical practice. Surgical workforce studies document a shortage of general surgeons, which is predicted to worsen, particularly in rural areas.

It is apparent that current surgery residency graduates report less confidence about their preparedness to enter surgical practice and their ability to independently perform many common procedures.[2] Some of this expressed lack of confidence may simply reflect a younger generation of surgeons who are more comfortable voicing their concerns. Fellowship program directors recently reported, however, that 30% of new fellows could not independently perform a laparoscopic cholecystectomy and 66% were not able to operate without direct supervision for 30 minutes of a major procedure.[3] Napolitano and associates[4] documented disparate findings concerning residency graduates' readiness for practice when comparing the opinions of young (≤45 years old) ACS fellows versus older (>45 years old) ACS fellows. Whereas 94% of younger surgeons thought that they had adequate surgical training and 91% felt prepared for surgical attending roles, only 59% of older surgeons believed that current surgical training was adequate and only 53% stated that graduates were prepared for the transition to surgical attending. Younger surgeons had concerns about business and practice skills during residency whereas older surgeons were troubled by paucity of training in communication, professionalism, and ethics during residency. In a survey of Southeastern Surgical Congress members, only 40% of respondents believed that new surgical graduates were sufficiently trained and could independently take call.[5]

Some investigators have opined that 80% of residency graduates opting for a subspecialty fellowship is further evidence that these young surgeons do not feel ready to enter practice.[6] This notion has been refuted by several recent studies of chief residents and new graduates in the United States and Canada in which the decision to pursue fellowship was rarely made on the basis of a sense of inadequate preparation for practice.[7,8] Furthermore, 2 studies have documented surprising graduate confidence regarding procedural skills.[8,9]

Although the magnitude of the problem of residency graduate confidence and preparedness for practice has not been definitively determined, it is clear that a subset of graduates each year does not feel confident in their abilities and does not feel ready for independent practice. It is likely that many more graduates have discomfort with some aspect(s) of the transition from training to practice. It is, therefore, incumbent on both surgical educators and senior surgeons in practice to develop effective programs to assist young surgeons in the early years of their practice with skills, such as operative judgment, practice management, running a clinic, communication, and work-life balance. This can be accomplished by personal mentoring, formal onboarding programs, or TTP educational experiences. In July 2012, the ACS Division of Education and the Accreditation Council for Graduate Medical Education cosponsored a conference to identify the most important issues surrounding the transition from surgical training to independent practice.[10] They developed the following recommendations based on analysis of the issues that were identified: (1) surgical residency should be redesigned with refocusing the curriculum using Surgical Council on Resident Education, additional use of simulation, competency-based assessment and advancement, and more robust operative skills assessment; (2) review of operative skills assessment and operative outcomes when hiring new graduates; (3) mentoring, preceptoring, and proctoring for new staff surgeons; (4) potential use of distance-learning capabilities for mentoring, preceptoring, and proctoring when necessary; and (5) development of additional milestones and entrustable professional activities to evaluate surgeons after training.

INSTITUTIONAL METHODS USED FOR TRANSITION FROM TRAINING TO SURGICAL PRACTICE

It has been shown that surgeons are most likely to leave their practices in the first 3 to 5 years.[11] Onboarding programs with monitoring of professional satisfaction, formalized mentoring, and development of leadership skills have been proposed to reduce surgeon attrition from academic medical centers.[11] Attending surgeon retention is much less costly in both human resource and financial terms than recruitment and training of yet another new surgeon. Most large university and independent medical centers include up to a week of mandatory orientation activities for new surgeons. Most of this time is spent on billing and coding instruction, compliance programs, information technology and electronic medical record training, credentialing, mandatory clinical training, physician compact/handbook review, meeting with key administrative staff, and campus orientation.

Although these quotidian activities are important, the keys to success for a new surgeon revolve around excellent communication, exercising sound clinical judgment in and out of the operating room, achieving good surgical outcomes, developing practice efficiency, and achieving a healthy work-life balance. The presence of an engaged senior mentor is an invaluable resource for a young surgeon who may be well trained but lack confidence or experience in some of these areas. Most senior partners provide guidance on an ad hoc basis; some provide more formal direction for their new colleagues. In the interest of patient safety and to allow a new partner to achieve a comfort level with operative cases, a senior partner may scrub on all procedures or a subset of more complex operations with a new partner for a period of time. How frequently this practice is applied is not known; it varies widely by institution and may be dependent on perceived skills of the new surgeon. In the survey of ACS fellows, younger surgeons reported that a senior partner assisted them on 9% of cases during the first year of practice; older surgeons estimated that they had scrubbed on 10% to 40% of operations performed by a new partner during the first year of practice.[4] In another survey of senior surgeons, it was estimated that 75% of new surgeons required assistance with elective cases and 82% with cases on call; however, operative assistance for a new partner was rarely (2%–3%) necessary after the first year of practice.[5] There is a great deal of variation based on the experience and confidence of the new partner as well as the interest in and commitment to mentoring or proctoring on the part of the senior partner.

Large academic medical centers and independent integrated health care systems have developed their own onboarding programs for new staff surgeons. Formal mentoring, career counseling, leadership training, and credentialing are common in university departments of surgery.[10] U.S. Armed Forces hospitals offer administrative and leadership training and intensive clinical experience in combat trauma for new graduates.[10] Integrated health care systems, such as Kaiser Permanente, require new physicians to study best practices and institutional care pathways.[10] In addition, at least 12 cases performed by new surgeons undergo departmental monitoring and review. The Kaiser Permanente health care system in San Diego assigns new surgeons to act as first assistants for senior surgeons and senior surgeons often scrub with new surgeons during the first 6 months of practice (Daniel Klaristenfeld, personal communication, 2015). A less formal program of mentoring is used at Geisinger Health System (Danville, PA, USA) and Gundersen Health System (La Crosse, WI, USA) in which new surgeons are assigned a senior mentor who provides guidance in establishing a new practice (John Widger, personal communication, 2015). Senior partners are available to scrub on more complex procedures or provide consultation in the operating room regarding decision making. At Gundersen Health System, surgical outcomes are tracked and reviewed at 6 and 12 months for all new surgical staff and ACS National Surgical Quality Improvement Program metrics are reviewed and compared for all general surgeons.

Program development for mentoring and proctoring is particularly problematic for new surgeons in solo practice or in isolated rural practice locations. Residency teaching faculty may be valuable resources for remote discussions of evaluation and management of difficult patients as well as advice on the business aspects of practice. Hands-on case proctoring is rarely practical from former mentors. Young surgeons in an isolated location may be able to rely on a more experienced surgeon in their region to scrub with them on more complex operations. The success of this activity depends on the willingness and availability of a colleague who must put a practice on hold to provide this generous service. Perhaps this mentoring and proctoring role would be a good activity for retired or part-time surgeons and could be organized by regional or national surgical organizations.

Murad and colleagues[12] at the University of Florida described a formal program to help neurosurgical trainees transition from residency to practice. Senior neurosurgery residents participated as fully mentored junior faculty members during the last 6 to 12 months of residency. The program included autonomous operative experience, practice management skill acquisition, an independent outpatient clinic and a critical review of patient outcomes. Less comprehensive TTP programs have been reported in other surgical specialties.[4,10] Most recently, the ACS has developed a formal TTP program that promises to be a valuable pathway for surgery residency graduates desiring additional experience to make a smooth transition into the practice of general surgery.[6,13]

THE AMERICAN COLLEGE OF SURGEONS TRANSITION TO PRACTICE GENERAL SURGERY PROGRAM

In 2012, the ACS, in conjunction with the American Board of Surgery, initiated a process to investigate development of a TTP program in general surgery to follow residency. The effort was intended to respond to concerns about residency graduates' readiness to enter practice, confidence in operative skills, lack of independence during training, and lack of exposure to a wide variety of cases. In addition, the worsening workforce shortage in general surgery was an additional motivation to enhance general surgery careers. The ACS TTP Steering Committee has been chaired by J. David Richardson from the University of the Louisville School of Medicine. After preliminary discussions and situation analysis, the ACS launched a 1-year TTP in general surgery program with the pilot testing of 6 sites in June 2013.[13] Key elements of this postresidency experience were trainee autonomy, personal mentoring by senior surgeons, graded clinical responsibility, flexible curriculum based on intake assessment of past experience and future goals, practice management skills acquisition, and clinical outcomes measurement. This program was not designed to be remedial in nature and it was not the intention of the ACS TTP Steering Committee that the program be considered a prerequisite for general surgery practice. It was recognized that graduates of many general surgery residencies are well prepared for general surgery practice and do not need this additional experience.[6]

Two TTP associates completed programs in 2014 and an additional 11 finished programs in 2015. There has been significant growth in the number of ACS TTP programs and the ACS has formalized the process of program accreditation. A list of guiding principles was recently approved to assist institutions in program development (**Box 1**). The foundational concepts remain senior mentorship, TTP associate autonomy and graded responsibility, flexible curriculum, practice management skill acquisition, and careful assessment with clinical outcomes analysis. Components of a robust practice management curriculum are listed in **Box 2**. As of April 2015, the ACS has approved 18 TTP programs (**Table 1**). This represents a diverse group of institutions, including university hospitals and independent health care systems with urban, suburban, and rural training sites.

The ACS recently convened a workshop to which TTP associates and program directors were invited. Strengths of the TTP experience enumerated by the TTP associates are listed in **Box 3**. Although all the TTP program directors remained enthusiastic about their TTP programs, several challenges for institutions and program directors were identified (**Box 4**). Realistic feedback from these experiences should inform the ACS and individual programs about further development or refinement.

FUTURE PREPARATION FOR SURGICAL PRACTICE

It is hoped that surgical education can change to better prepare tomorrow's residency graduates for either general surgery practice or subspecialty fellowships.[8,14] More practice management skills must be infused into the curriculum of all surgical residencies.[15,16] Earlier exposure to surgical procedures, efficient use of simulation technology, and competency-based procedure evaluation may improve operative proficiency. Progressive autonomy may be possible using entrustable professional

---

Box 1
Guiding principles for American College of Surgeons transition to practice programs

1. Dedicated TTP program chief should provide leadership, supervision, and quality oversight for the program.

2. One or more TTP senior associates in full-time surgical practice should serve as clinical mentors.

3. The TTP program must not interfere with the training of residents and fellows at the sponsoring institution.

4. A flexible curriculum with progressive responsibility/autonomy should be designed around the TTP associate to result in a well-balanced general surgery experience.

5. An intake assessment of the TTP associate's past experience and future career goals should be performed to design an individualized curriculum congruent with TTP associate needs.

6. An autonomous outpatient clinic experience with opportunities for graded responsibility must be provided.

7. A robust curriculum in practice management skills is required.

8. Outcomes of cases performed by the TTP associate must be tracked and reviewed – preferably using the ACS Surgeon Specific Registry.

9. Periodic formative and summative assessments must be completed by teaching faculty to evaluate TTP associate performance.

10. Periodic assessments of teaching faculty performance must be completed by the TTP associate.

11. The TTP program budget must be sufficient to cover program and associate costs.

12. Salary and benefits to include professional liability insurance with tail coverage, vacation, and continuing medical education programs must be supplied by the sponsoring institution.

---

activities and credentialing during residency.[14] If these and other changes were universally adopted by all residencies in an optimal educational environment, then formal TTP programs might not be necessary. In the meantime, it remains to be seen if the ACS TTP in general surgery programs will gain traction among candidates as well as residency program directors.

Box 2
Components of practice management curriculum

1. Billing and coding

2. Reimbursement principles

3. Contract negotiations

4. Professional liability insurance

5. Medical liability case preparation

6. Patient scheduling

7. Insurance preauthorization and billing

8. Quality improvement processes

9. Patient safety initiatives

10. Retirement planning

Table 1
Approved American College of Surgeons transition to practice programs as of April 2015

	Health System	Location
1	Kaiser Permanente – San Diego	San Diego, CA
2	University of Florida/St. Vincent's Health System	Jacksonville, FL
3	Mercer University School of Medicine	Macon, GA
4	University of Louisville School of Medicine	Louisville, KY
5	Louisiana State University – Shreveport	Shreveport, LA
6	Anne Arundel Medical Center	Annapolis, MD
7	Montefiore Medical Center	Bronx, NY
8	Carolinas Medical Center	Charlotte, NC
9	Wake Forest School of Medicine	Winston-Salem, NC
10	Ohio State University College of Medicine	Columbus, OH
11	Geisinger Health System	Danville, PA
12	Alpert Medical School of Brown University	Providence, RI
13	Medical University of South Carolina	Charleston, SC
14	University of Tennessee College of Medicine	Chattanooga, TN
15	University of Texas Health Science Center at San Antonio	San Antonio, TX
16	Mid-Atlantic Permanente Medical Group	McLean, VA
17	Eastern Virginia Medical School	Norfolk, VA
18	Gundersen Health System	La Crosse, WI

Regardless of the success of TTP programs, graduates of surgical residencies and fellowships will always require a period of adjustment as they transform from trainees to experienced surgeons. An effective method of making this a smooth transition is important for patient safety, success and retention of the new surgeon, and stability for mature practices. Larger health care systems should be able to develop effective in-house onboarding programs with attentive, proactive mentoring and case proctoring/supervision to allow a safe transition from trainee to staff surgeon. Small, isolated surgical practices may need to rely on outside mentoring and supervision or video-based case reviews to accomplish the same goal. National and regional surgical societies may be in a position to facilitate this process in states with many remote practices.

Box 3
Transition to practice program strengths highlighted by transition to practice associates

1. Autonomy/independence with safety net provided by TTP senior associates
2. Flexible curriculum to meet individual needs of the TTP associate
3. New technical skill acquisition
4. Mentoring relationship provided by the TTP senior associates
5. Clinical and procedural opportunities to build confidence
6. Independent outpatient clinic experience with "own patients"
7. Ability to practice with continuity of care
8. Chance to learn and use practice management skills

Box 4
Challenges encountered by institutions sponsoring American College of Surgeons transition to practice programs

1. Competition for cases with other learners
2. Competition for cases with new surgical faculty
3. Less program acceptance by multiple surgical specialists who must provide training.
4. Less autonomy/independence on short specialty rotations
5. Difficult to provide graded responsibility over short time frames
6. Perception from potential applicants and residency program directors that TTP programs are "remedial" programs
7. Credentialing issues: Are TTP associates trainees or junior faculty? What are credentialing ramifications for reported performance concerns during these experiences?
8. Steep learning curve for the TTP associate to accommodate to new institution/health care system/electronic medical record

---

REFERENCES

1. Lewis FR, Klingensmith ME. Issues in general surgery residency training – 2012. Ann Surg 2012;256:553–9.
2. Bucholz EM, Sue GR, Yeo H, et al. Our trainees' confidence: results from a national survey of 4136 US general surgery residents. Arch Surg 2011;146:907–14.
3. Mattar SG, Alseidi AA, Jones DB, et al. General surgery residency inadequately prepares trainees for fellowship: results of a survey of fellowship program directors. Ann Surg 2013;258:440–9.
4. Napolitano LM, Savarise M, Paramo JC, et al. Are general surgery residents ready to practice? A survey of the American College of Surgeons Board of Governors and Young Fellows Association. J Am Coll Surg 2014;218:1063–72.
5. Nakayama DK, Taylor SM. SESC Practice Committee survey: surgical practice in the duty-hour restriction era. Am Surg 2013;79:711–5.
6. Richardson JD. ACS transition to practice program offers residents additional opportunities to hone skills. Bull Am Coll Surg 2013;98:23–7.
7. Nadler A, Ashamalla S, Escallon J, et al. Career plans and perceptions in readiness to practice of graduating general surgery residents in Canada. J Surg Educ 2015;72:205–11.
8. Klingensmith ME, Cogbill TH, Luchette F, et al. Factors influencing the decision of surgery residency graduates to pursue general surgery practice versus fellowship. Ann Surg 2015;262(3):449–55.
9. Friedell ML, VanderMeer TJ, Cheatham ML, et al. Perceptions of graduating general surgery chief residents: are they confident in their training? J Am Coll Surg 2014;218:695–703.
10. Sachdeva AK, Flynn TC, Brigham TP, et al, American College of Surgeons (ACS) Division of Education, Accreditation Council for Graduate Medical Education (ACGME). Interventions to address challenges associated with the transition from residency training to independent surgical practice. Surgery 2014;155:867–82.
11. Satiani B, Williams TE, Brod H, et al. A review of trends in attrition rates for surgical faculty: a case for a sustainable retention strategy to cope with demographic and economic realities. J Am Coll Surg 2013;216:944–53.

12. Murad GJ, Lister JR, Friedman WA, et al. Enhancing competence in graduates through a transition to practice program in neurological surgery. Clin Neurosurg 2010;57:141–4.
13. Hoyt DB. Looking forward. Bull Am Coll Surg 2013;98:7–10.
14. Cogbill TH. Surgical education and training: how are they likely to change? J Am Coll Surg 2015;220:1032–5.
15. Jones K, Lebron RA, Mangram A, et al. Practice management education during surgical residency. Am J Surg 2008;196:878–81.
16. Klingensmith ME, Cogbill TH, Samonte K, et al. Practice administration training needs of recent general surgery graduates. Surgery 2015;158(3):773–6.

Alternative Considerations for Surgical Training and Funding

Ronald F. Martin, MD[a,b,c],*

KEYWORDS

- Surgical training • Funding • Graduate medical education • Alternatives

KEY POINTS

- The system of training we use is a minimally modified version of the training systems that were established in the United States in the 1880s.
- The current system of graduate medical education (GME) training we have is paid for largely by federal monies and subjected to oversight of the Accreditation Council for Graduate Medical Education in order to qualify for that financial support; general surgeons are certified by a monolithic certification system.
- Changes in clinical team structure and incorporation of our current GME system into a life-long continuing medical education system within our clinical care environments could give us opportunities to greater diversify the surgical workforce and better distribute the costs of surgical training.

INTRODUCTION

Since the late 1880s surgical residency programs have existed in forms that are similar to our current models. Many important variations have been introduced over time including; transition from an open-ended to time based training models, transition from the pyramidal to the rectangular model, recognition as a national concern during the creation of Medicare including a shift to substantial federal funding, and the creation and modification of work hours regulations from 2003 to present, to name but a few. The distinct model of a medical student who transitions to resident or fellow as student/employee who then finally transitions to independent staff surgeon has been the standard model as well. We have assessed adequacy of training largely by national testing processes such as those offered by the American Board of Surgery

[a] Marshfield Clinic and Saint Joseph's Hospital, 1000 North Oak Avenue, Marshfield, WI 54449, USA; [b] Department of Surgery, University of Wisconsin School of Medicine and Public Health, 750 Highland Avenue, Madison, WI 53726, USA; [c] United States Army Reserve, Medical Corps, USA
* Marshfield Clinic and Saint Joseph's Hospital, 1000 North Oak Avenue, Marshfield, WI 54449.
E-mail address: rmartin@yorkhospital.com

Surg Clin N Am 96 (2016) 35–46
http://dx.doi.org/10.1016/j.suc.2015.09.002
0039-6109/16/$ – see front matter © 2016 Elsevier Inc. All rights reserved.

since its creation in 1937. On aggregate this system has worked remarkably well though as economic, demographic, and cultural changes continue to evolve, one must wonder if we were to change our models how might we do that and what reasoning could we use. This article's focus will be to take a stratospheric view of what could be done, particularly in the United States, rather than characterize what happens in other countries with other health economic systems.

DISCLAIMERS

By way of full disclosure, I have made my living for the past nine years as a program director of a categorical general surgery training program. My salary during that time was largely, though not entirely, supported by funds paid to our sponsoring institutions by the Center for Medicare and Medicaid Services (CMS). I am board certified and re-certified in surgery by the American Board of Surgery (ABS). I have served as an Associate Examiner for the Certifying Exam (CE) for the ABS on multiple occasions and serve as an examination consultant question writer for American Board of Surgery In-Training Exam (ABSITE). I have been a member of multiple state and national committees of the American College of Surgeons (ACS) including the joint group on Transition to Practice jointly sponsored by the ACS and Accreditation Council for Graduate Medical Education (ACGME). I have also served as the Designated Institutional Officer (DIO) for our institution as well as Chairman of the Graduate Medical Education Committee (GMEC). Lastly, I served as Associate Dean for the Medical School (an Association of American Medical Colleges (AAMC) approved school) with which we are affiliated. I greatly respect and admire those with whom I have worked and in no way question their qualifications, ethics, or dedication to what they have done. The views expressed in this article, except where directly attributed to a specific source, are solely my own and do not necessarily reflect the views of any of the organizations listed above or otherwise described within the context of this document nor do my views necessarily represent the views of the United States Army, Department of Defense, or United States Government.

FURTHER DISCLAIMER AND EDITORIAL NOTE

The *Surgical Clinics of North America* nearly exclusively publishes material that reviews the existing literature and adds expert perspective and context to our understanding of that body of knowledge. In this issue we are attempting to review issues that span the arc of a surgeon's career from medical school through to retirement. From an editorial standpoint for this issue we felt compelled to also consider ideas that might be outside of current experience to at least stimulate a discussion of paths we might regard that are not simply tweaks of the system we already use. The ideas that are expressed in this article represent considerations that to the best of our knowledge have not been tried. The basis for these proposals come from identifying limitations of our current models encountered during decades of experience in having to solve typical and atypical problems involving both the training of resident and staff surgeons, as well as addressing labor and business issues of small and large medical corporations and/or developing medical capability in austere wartime environments. The concepts given for consideration are speculative by their very nature.

Much of what will follow in this article may be interpreted as a suggestion for complete change in process for the development of surgeons. It is meant to provide alternative constructs to what we are currently doing rather than list condemnations of what we have done. These ideas are not delivered as "tested methods" of what would work better but rather to stimulate thought about what might work better. I hope it is viewed in that light.

CURRENT STATUS

The education of a surgeon as with all other forms of education has evolved and changed since the beginning of recorded time. Despite much of the hand wringing and condemnations of past practices that we sometimes hear, we are left with one indisputable conclusion: the system as it has evolved has created a powerfully capable surgical workforce. It would be difficult to imagine that a continuation of the current system or continued slow evolution would not continue to create excellent physicians. However, it is not unreasonable to consider whether changes, either large or small, would better address the training of surgeons and the delivery of care to those who depend on them.

When one is contemplating making change, it is always best to understand what the current state of affairs actually is. Describing the entire history of surgical education is well beyond the scope of this article; thus, the discussion is confined to the highlights of surgical training in the United States. Halsted is credited with creating the first surgical residency program in the United States in 1889. Of note, it was pyramidal and there was no guarantee when or if one would complete training.[1] Dr Edward Churchill of Massachusetts General Hospital (MGH) made the first major change to residency structure by creating a rectangular-structured program that was different not only in the proportion of people who would finish but also how long it would take to do so. In the modified structure, 6 residents entered, 4 of whom would do 4 years of training (considered sufficient to learn surgery at the time) and 2 of whom would train for an additional 2 years in order to become a professor or stay on staff at MGH.[2,3] Of note Churchill was reported to have been opposed to the fixed length of time for a surgical residency, as it did not allow "latitude for interests and proficiencies."[3] The basic rectangular structure set forth by Dr Churchill at MGH has lasted more or less to this day for all our existing general surgery training programs, though in the latter part of the twentieth century calls for changes for flexibility and focused became more prominent.[4]

Regulation and oversight of training programs has also evolved over time. Following the Flexner report in 1910, new focus on recognizing and improving the quality of health care education developed. A Federation of State Medical Boards was created in 1912, and the American Medical Association published a list of hospitals approved to educate interns in 1914. By 1927, the American College of Surgeons published standards for graduate training in surgery, and the American Board of Surgery was founded 1937.[1] Graduate medical education (GME) and funding increased to the level of national debate with the creation of Medicare in the 1960s, and in 1972 the Liaison Committee for Graduate Medical Education was formed that later was renamed as the Accreditation Council for Graduate Medical Education (ACGME). The Residency Review Committees, which predate the ACGME, are now under the regulatory umbrella of the ACGME.

The amount and sources of funding available for GME is difficult to assess with extreme accuracy given the myriad of sources that are involved and the sheer complexity of the systems involved. That said, we can get at least in the ballpark. In a report from the Institute of Medicine on GME financing, estimates of federal spending on GME range from $12 to $14 million per year.[5] This estimate includes funds from Medicare, Medicaid, Veterans Health Administration, and the Health Resources and Services Administration (HRSA). Other sources of funding, such as the Department of Defense, private insurers, other private institutional or philanthropic sources, and other state funding, are not included in their report.[5] Data provided by the Center for Medicare and Medicaid Services (CMS) state that total US health care expenditures for 2103 reached $2.9 trillion, or approximately 17.4% of the gross domestic product.[6] This amount would place total federal spending on GME at approximate 0.5% of all health care spending in the United States. With that review in mind, we can start to consider options. As always, a high yield place to start is to follow the money.

ALTERNATIVE FUNDING STRATEGIES

One of the major stumbling blocks to reform and progress in the training of surgical residents is the current mechanism of funding. Dollars provided from federal sources to sponsoring institutions are completely contingent on the sponsoring institution being accredited by the ACGME and compliant with ACGME rules and regulations. Although most of the rules and regulations that an institution are subject to are quite reasonable, some are simply either impractical for surgeons in training or actually counterproductive. Independent of one's views on any of the specific rules or requirements, one fact remains inescapable: if we did not depend on CMS dollars, then we would not necessarily have to train surgical residents under the ACGME rules. This concept, of course, causes panic in some who use CMS dollars to pay the salaries of residents who in turn supply work (service) to offset difficulties achieving a satisfactory economic bottom line in clinical service delivery. The panic relates to the question: where else would the money come from? Although that may be a good question for some, it is also somewhat irrelevant. The better questions are as follows: should the US citizens be financially responsible for making training institutions more economically viable by underwriting surgical resident (or other trainee for that matter) education through the tax code? And should those organizations be able to benefit economically from a commodity created by using taxpayer dollars?

Training Costs

Let us look at the costs of training first. The more tangible costs of training surgical residents are the salary and benefits that they receive, plus the cost of insuring them for liability and other education-related expenses. Some of the other costs relate to the cost of paying faculty, whether through direct compensation or other means; the cost of administering programs and institutions; the costs of compliance with a myriad of extra rules; and some difficult-to-calculate costs for offsets in individual practitioner and institutional efficiencies. Of course these costs are offset by whatever services the trainee can provide that either create value-added services that are otherwise reimbursed, freeing up others to engage in lucrative activities, or reducing the potential for lost revenue or penalties when problems are headed off. There is also the benefit of professional satisfaction and fulfillment in developing the new generation of thinkers and practitioners. There are benefits to creating the new workforce, though the training institutions do not solely enjoy these benefits. There may be philanthropic opportunities that may directly offset expenses that are uniquely associated with training environments. All in all, though, I suspect most program directors will assure you that their institution probably pays more to educate residents than it receives. What may be less agreed on is whether the net negative on the balance sheet is offset by the other services that did not have to be purchased in lieu of trainee effort. In one report by Meara and colleagues,[7] the cost to the institution of supporting GME surgical training was calculated at more than $6000 per resident per year. The author's institutional contribution per resident is higher than that.

Cost of Graduate Medical Education As a Function of the Larger Economy

The amount of money spent on GME by the federal government is actually fairly trivial compared with the overall cost of health care in the United States. To briefly recap, roughly $12 to $14 billion is paid to training programs annually. That might seem like a large sum but compared with the roughly $2.9 trillion spent annually on health care in the United States, it represents slight less than 0.5% of all health care dollars spent. On a grand scale we would be fine in the health care industry if we had to absorb a 0.5% cut across the board; but under the current structure, such an even absorption of loss across the entire spectrum of health care is not what would happen. Most of the health care in the United States is delivered in medial environments that are not involved in GME training, so none of those facilities would see a direct loss if the federal GME money went away. Training centers would, however, suffer disproportionate losses. Furthermore, the more dependent on trainee service for labor supply an organization is, the worse it would suffer the cessation of federal money. This point raises 2 concerns: training centers benefit disproportionately from federal money to supply labor and nontraining environments bear none of the cost of developing the people from whom they will eventually financially benefit. The former concern is further muddied by the fact that leaders of the organizations who benefit most from federal dollars for training also serve in most of the positions in national surgical leadership who interact with government, providing at least the potential for a conflict of interest when they represent the surgical community as whole.

Resident Training As a Commodity

If we take a step back and look at residency training as something other than an educational stepping-stone, perhaps alternatives become available. For instance, let us consider GME as a process that creates a commodity, which it does. Also, let us consider that commodity has a value, which it does, and then the assessment of the cost of training changes. First we have to consider the value of the raw material—interns mostly in this example. The monetary value of an intern in terms of delivering work is pretty minimal really, but it does exist. Subtract from that the level of debt that that person has incurred to achieve his or her initial state of usefulness and you have some sense of the commodity value of a new intern. Even though that value is likely to be substantially negative, the potential for value is what matters. The more trained a resident becomes, the more that he or she can do that will either lead to increasing the efficiency of delivering billable services or serving on a team to increase team efficiency. By the time a resident completes training, he or she can step into roles that require less or no supervision and can provide services that are directly compensated or indirectly compensated through facilities' fees and so forth. Eventually, most surgeons enter into gainful employment that allows them to practice and repay their indebtedness from education as well as make a substantial surplus over their careers and prepare for retirement. Of course there are exceptions, but the rule is still valid. If the rule is valid, then one point becomes inviolate: creating a surgeon as a commodity is an investment with a positive return, likely a highly positive return. A derivative concept, therefore, is that creating a surgeon (or transforming from a graduated medical student into a surgeon) is a value-adding step and is worthy of compensation.

One form of compensating for the value addition mentioned is the current system we have: direct monetary compensation from federal funding and time/effort trade-off for faculty in lieu of effort performed by trainees. In my opinion, that dislocates the cost-benefit equation of training quality and effort. The government pays, and those of us in training take the money and benefit to whatever degree we do on a transactional basis limited to the duration of training. The subsequent employing environments and the surgeon in training share the long-term financial reward. That system is actually okay in many regards, but it is also lacking. Its main failure is it does not hold the right people to the right responsibilities for assuring the quality of the commodity along the way. Medical schools can dislocate what they charge from the quality of the student whom they graduate (a topic well beyond the scope of what can be addressed in this article). Residency and other GME programs also can finish people who may be more or less valuable than others independent of what we get reimbursed for in the process. Lastly, surgeons and the organizations that hire them are largely responsible for long-term investment in the development of quality and value and are increasingly responsible for correcting deficiencies in the product they initially acquire. The costs are always front-loaded, and the last consumer always bears the responsibility for correcting deficiencies.

Alternatively, though, we could consider something very different. Let us consider that that phase of training between medical school and practice is a product in and of itself to be sold. We could sell it to the trainee; that would be called tuition. Although that argument could be made, I think it would be stillborn in today's economic market. Most people coming out of medical school are sufficiently in debt that further deferring income production and increasing debt for multiple years would be a nonstarter on the grand scale. We could, however, defer the cost and provide supplemental income to be recouped at a later time. For example, we could pay a resident a salary of $150,000 per year while he or she was a resident with $50,000 being the base salary and $100,000 being advanced compensation. Also, we could agree that on graduation, the advanced compensation would either have to be worked off as an employee of the training institution or be paid off either by the surgeon or an acquiring company that would employ the surgeon. The specific numbers listed are not relevant but are simplified for example. Such a scheme would do several things. First, it would allow the trainee to repay any previous educational debt at an accelerated pace. Second, it would make the training program more directly accountable for producing a quality product that was worth a future employer paying to acquire the contract. It would also make the training program desirous of producing a high-quality surgeon because the default would be to repay the cost of training by employing the surgeon directly. Lastly, it would diffuse the overall cost of training to all components of health care delivery because every entity that employs surgeons would eventually have to pay some cost for acquiring practitioners. The net result would be to diffuse the costs of training surgeons among all payer sources, including the government through Medicare and Medicaid, the private insurance payers, the self-payers, and any other revenue source. Also, if economic theory holds true, it would make the hirers of new surgeons more demanding and critical of the product they acquired, thus, forcing training programs to reconsider their training practices and standards.

The process of transitioning to such a payment/compensation model would present issues, but in the long run the benefits would probably outweigh the costs and difficulties. Such a model would place the accountability and reward for training at the same level. It would also put training environments in a position to more carefully consider the quality of medical school graduates or trainees that they desire and recruit. It would allow those of us who claim we know better what conditions under which to train surgeons (and we do claim that) to do so without being beholden to the current level of regulation by the ACGME. We would all have to deliver better training and surgeon product rather than rely on reputation to succeed if we had economic skin in the game for substandard training.

The up-front costs of doing this would be substantial: at least $12 to $14 billion dollars if we are actually using the current federal funding we receive for what it is intended. Given the overall economic return on investment for creating the average surgeon, it is reasonable to expect that we could find private, or even public, funding partners to work with us to get the system running. Also, as in other matters of public need, there is nothing to prohibit local, regional, state, or federal programs from providing funds on the back end to allocate surgical resources to areas of high need with marginal resources. Such an alteration in funding from beginning of training to completion of training would, however, allow public spending for types of training to address areas of greater need rather than front-load spending and subsidize training in areas that are already adequately resourced. This change could have the added benefit of addressing the distribution, or misdistribution, side of the problem with critical surgical access in some areas. Lastly, if we couple the funding changes with modification of training paradigms, then we can even better tailor delivering surgical capability to our communities, which brings us to the next topic: what surgeons need to know.

CERTIFICATION DRIVES TRAINING MODELS

According to the American Board of Surgery's "Booklet of Information,"[8] residency training in general surgery requires experience in all of the following content areas in order to be admissible for examination leading to board certification: alimentary tract (including bariatric surgery), abdomen and its contents, breast, skin and soft tissue, endocrine system, solid organ transplantation, pediatric surgery, surgical critical care, surgical oncology (including head and neck surgery), trauma/burns and emergency surgery, and vascular surgery. Although it is a lofty goal to have all trained general surgeons achieve this experience and have all accredited programs manage to provide some kind of training education that meets these goals, we have to ask: is it necessary? If there is a surgeon out in practice in the United States who actually does all of the listed components of general surgery or even a substantial fraction, I am not aware of that person. I absolutely agree that exposure to all these areas of training can be extremely helpful when one finds himself or herself isolated from other resources. I can personally attest that in austere environments, such as I found myself in in Iraq and Afghanistan, a broad-based surgical education was useful. However, in the less austere clinical environments within North America, including rural environments, one almost never finds oneself in a position where there is neither additional local resources available nor the ability to transfer a patient to a more greatly resourced environment. Although there will always be a few exceptions that one could point to, we cannot and should not build a system to handle extreme outlier exceptions. So this begs the question: why such a broad required experience for ABS certification? Also, should certification be modular or monolithic?

There are many good arguments for monolithic training models and certification. One board is easier to manage and oversee than many boards or subboards. One board certification provides a broader-based certified surgeon who can fill multiple needs. Global retesting and recertifying requires fewer processes than multiple modular recertifications. Even if all that were stipulated to be true, it probably pales in strength to one counterargument: nobody, or virtually nobody, actually does all the things ABS certification states one is certified to do.

The arguments for modular certification are pretty much the opposite as for monolithic certification. One would only certify in areas in which they practiced. One would not need to spend time reviewing or relearning material solely for the sake of taking an examination that will not alter one's practice patterns. More focused certification may lead to certifying examinations actually having greater credibility on assuring quality practitioners.

It is a quite difficult to make the argument that my junior partner who has a practice based exclusively on breast surgery and provides no coverage to general surgery colleagues should require the current monolithic recertification by the ABS. It is just as difficult to make the argument that a trauma surgeon needs to be tested on endocrine surgery or a surgical oncologist benefits from being tested on the principles of trauma and burn surgery. Even if we move away from the aforementioned component-related issues, let us examine something like endoscopy. The ABS has added a requirement that all graduates of accredited general surgery programs who complete their residency training in the 2017 to 2018 academic year will be required to show completion of the Fundamentals of Endoscopic Surgery (FES) curriculum. This latest requirement was added by the ABS despite the fact that at the 2015 Association of Program Directors in Surgery's (APDS) annual meeting representatives of the ABS informed us that only approximately 20% of ABS-certified surgeons practice any form of endoscopy (direct communication, breakout sessions on FES, APDS annual meeting, Seattle, Washington, 2015). This figure implies that 80% of graduates of categorical training programs will now have to take a high-stakes examination for something they will not do in clinical practice, at their or their program's expense, in order to become admissible to the ABS qualifying examination. Although this preserves monolithic certification, it really begs the question of whether this best certifies the surgeon or protects the public interest.

On the other hand, one can certainly make the argument that broad-based surgical training confers certain benefits to all who practice surgery: one develops a greater skill set by learning from multiple disciplines and subdisciplines, is better able to communicate with other surgical disciplines when patients require poly-disciplinary care, and is better able to communicate with other surgeons when handing off care to someone with a differing specialty. All that being accepted as true, is it worth the redundancy of effort and expense in training every surgeon that way? And if one feels that initial certification may require this very broad training experience, should it be the standard for recertification?

One of the more commonly used arguments for maintaining monolithic surgical certification is the need to maintain broad-based certification to address the shortage of general surgeons in the United States. Modular certification would further reduce the number of trained general surgeons in remote areas. This argument is a little hard to support. One problem with the construct is that we do not really have a definition of what a general surgeon is. Frequently one sees comparison of numbers of general surgeons in practice now compared with the numbers of general surgeons practicing in the late 1980s. I suggest we agree that premise is nonstarter. In the late 1980s, general surgeons did the lion's share of thoracic, vascular, oncologic, foregut, hepatopancreaticobiliary, breast, colorectal, and trauma surgery and wound care. Although it is really difficult to get exact data, it seems likely that if we included all the specialties that currently cover work previously done by general surgeons and added those who currently hold themselves out to be general surgeons, we would probably have a significant increase in surgical capacity compared with the late 1980s. That is not to say that we would not have a shortage of surgical capacity for the needs of today. It does, however, raise the question of how much of our shortages are due to inadequate numbers of surgeons and how much is related to the distribution of surgical capacity. Most likely the answer will be some of both. The solution to the absolute number part of the problem is to train more people, whereas the answer to the distribution problem may be generating greater capacity of those who are in lower-demand environments. That is where modular certification perhaps has its greatest potential. We already see the use of general surgeons to provide endoscopic capability in areas where there are limited gastroenterology resources. Adding modular certification for some orthopedic, obstetric, head and neck conditions, as well as other areas may make it more efficient to keep some resources local in austere environments. That said, adding on capability in one area of someone's practice usually means subtracting it in another. Customizing capability to local needs by modular certification may be a solution to disparate local needs. It may also decrease the amount of time required to train someone to serve the local needs of a community, which brings us to the next point: how long should we take to train a general surgeon?

LENGTH OF TRAINING FOR GENERAL SURGERY

The idea of 5 years being the appropriate length of time to train a general surgeon is pretty arbitrary when one really thinks about it. Going back to the first time-bounded residencies established by Churchill, the fixed length was questioned.[2] If one wants proof its arbitrary, then all one has to do is consider the years 2003 and 2014. In each of those years the ACGME implemented changes that would curtail the amount of time residents could spend working per week, effectively reducing their training opportunity exposure per week; but we did not increase the number of weeks of training per year or the number of years of training. We still considered 5 years the correct length of time to train a surgeon. One has to wonder why not change the length of training. Were we overtraining surgeons beforehand? It is doubtful. Did we become more efficient in our training afterward? That is also doubtful, yet at least one could try to make the argument that better-rested residents are more efficient learners. Sadly, every metric we have that might showed improved learning with diminished work hour requirements, such as the ABS qualifying examination and certifying examination results does not bear that out. In fact performance on these exams declined to the point that the ABS modified the examinations as a response. So why not change? The most plausible explanation goes back to money. Training institutions receive federal funding for residents on a per-year basis. If we increased the number of years of training per residency program, then we would effectively increase the amount of money the federal government would need to spend on at least the direct medical expenditure portion of GME, assuming they continued to support residency training at similar dollar levels per year. If general surgery training only increased by 1 year to offset the diminished learning opportunity per week, we would need at least a 20% increase in federal spending or the extra costs would have to be absorbed by the training institutions. Alternatively, we could have reduced the amount of spending per resident per year; but, as mentioned earlier, that would unlikely be acceptable to students graduating from medical school with increasing amounts of educational debt. So the most likely reason we decreased work hours but did not increase years of training was political: it is revenue neutral for the government and incoming residents could make the previously expected pay for fewer hours worked, thus, leaving only the institutions to financially suffer by getting less service from residents for the same amount of money. Couple the aforementioned information with the a shift in focus for resident training to be educational over service, though both are quite related in many cases, and the institutions are left without a significant political argument to garner sympathy for their being wronged.

Although economics and politics might explain why we did not change the length of training after the work hours restrictions became part of our culture, they do not address the correctness of the length to begin with. The length of 5 years is most likely a historical accident of sorts. The introduction of a residency program as previously described was in response to moving away from apprenticeships. It is most likely that then as now most people learn at different rates and are ready to accept different level of responsibilities at different rates. There have to be natural boundaries to lengths of training that are both learner and training system dependent; too short of a period of time and the learner cannot be exposed to enough material and the instructors do not have enough time to assess consistency of performance and too long of a period of time and both the learner and the instructors are wasting one another's time and valuable resources. Knowing that these boundaries exist is easy, but knowing what the boundaries should be is not easy.

When a chef was asked how long to cook something I heard him reply, "You cook it until it is done." It is difficult to argue with such logic. So when is a surgeon done? When he or she can do what he or she has to do safely and efficiently. The amount of time for that to take place is highly likely to be variable and dependent on the learner, the instructors, the number of patients one encounters, the depth and breadth of clinical problems to be addressed, and a long list of less tangible variables. Suffice it to say it will be variable. Historically, we eschewed assessment of an individual trainee's readiness because there was too arbitrary of a nature to the assessment and/or it was too much work to do it correctly. That is probably still true to some degree, so we are left with the conundrum of how to solve the puzzle. That brings us to our last topic.

DO AWAY WITH RESIDENCY TRAINING AS WE KNOW IT

This last topic may be difficult for some readers. I apologize. Let me suggest we do away with residency training as we know it. Now some of you may think of this as a murder of sorts, but allow me to defend myself: it was dead when I found it.

Allow me to back up slightly. If residency training were a viable concept in the here and now, we would not worry about its length, its completeness, its ability to turn out a globally functional surgeon, or the economics of training. As previously mentioned, all of the factors are concerns and have been for a very long time. We have been running a code on general surgery residency training for decades (at least) and its time to call: time of death: some time ago already. Residency died of a disease of self-delusion, and that delusion can be summed up in one word: autonomy.

On the national level, we have been banging the drum of *we must restore autonomy* in the lament of our surgical training decline. It has been opined that if we just give our residents more autonomy, they will be as awesome as we were. There are 2 main problems with that argument: the first is that there was never any real autonomy to restore, and the second is that we were not that awesome. Surgeons may have been great leaders, may have been great innovators, and may have been great clinicians; but they were never autonomous. If you want to test this, see how successful you are at operating on patients who are not anesthetized or tying knots and removing your own clamps. See if your postoperative instructions get followed without a nurse or your prescriptions get filled without a pharmacist. It should not take too long to figure out that we surgeons are part of teams; nearly by definition we are not autonomous. So please let us finally let that concept go.

If one is willing to take heed to my suggestion to abandon the idea that we surgeons are autonomous, then we start to get the idea that we really do not need residency training as we know it. After all, residency training is really a lower-paid combination of a student/employee position that is a spacer between the concept of medical student and autonomous surgeon; rid us of the latter and we do not really need residency training. Instead we need to make people functioning members of the team. That is not equivalent to saying that graduating medical students do not need additional training, they do as do we all over the entirety of our career.

If we combine the observation of all the earlier sections in this article and the logic incorporated into each, perhaps we can create a model that could be an alternative to what we are currently doing. First, let us leave the CMS, HRSA, and other federal money out of the front end of training. After all, it is not that much money, as a percentage of health care spending, and it comes with far too many strings attached. Second, let us move to not just modular certification but also stratified certification (more on that shortly). Lastly, let us move those who would have been residents into the clinical teams and incorporate their services and educational requirements into the clinical elements of organizations that have the capacity to develop talent. We would not be the only professionals to do this; in fact we might be late to the game. Lawyers, bankers, the military, and even the clergy already do it and have been for a very long time.

If we were to focus on taking medical students after graduating and giving them training and opportunities to play the various positions on the team while gaining formal education before allowing them to be significant supervisors or top-tier leaders, perhaps we might be better off. We could remediate gaps in undergraduate medical education (though we should not have to) and provide testing and certification of basic fundamental milestones before allowing junior colleagues to engage in independent billable services. We could create metrics to be met in terms of documented experience as well as fact-based and judgment-based training and assessment before one could advance to providing less supervised care and greater supervision of junior personnel. We could allow greater flexibility in training/work schedules to reflect the variable needs of addressing other personal goals, such as having children or dealing with other family issues, something historically we do not have a great track record for. We could allow more tailoring of acquisition of advanced or additional skill sets to meet local and regional needs not just for those who would be in the current training window but also for those who need to incorporate new technology or knowledge, or simply refresh, into their practices at any time during one's career. We do not have to look too far in the rearview mirror to see how helpful that could have been with new technology, such as videoscopic surgery.

We could use the board certification for initial certification with or without modular modification. Perhaps we could use modular certification for recertification and/or maintenance of certification. Take it a step further and we could use actual quality and outcomes data and indication/utilization review for maintenance of certification. If you really want to make life easier push for either federal medical licensing or absolute reciprocity between states for medical licensing and mandatory transfer of all state verifications of medical practitioner information to the Federal Credentials Verification Service. If we were serious about protecting patients instead of fiefdoms, we would have done that already.

The National Labor Relations Board may have ruled that residents were both students and employees, but in reality so are fellows and attending surgeons. To artificially separate one group of worker-learners (residents) from another group of people who are also worker-learners (fellows and staff surgeons) one does at one's own peril. The introduction and emphasis of lifelong learning has blurred the distinction between resident, fellow, or staff surgeon to the point of irrelevance.

SUMMARY

The system of training we use is a minimally modified version of the training systems that were established in the United States in the 1880s. The current system of GME training we have is paid for largely by federal monies and subjected to oversight of the ACGME in order to qualify for that financial support. General surgeons are certified by a monolithic certification system. Changes in clinical team structure and incorporation of our current GME system into a lifelong continuing medical education system within our clinical care environments could give us opportunities to greater diversify the surgical workforce and better distribute the costs of surgical training. Although moving funding to the completion of training and incorporating residency training into the standard workforce environments may seem radical to some, it does not change the goals of what we currently do; in fact, it may advance some of them. Getting the right patient to the right people in the right place with the right resources at the right time is how we improve quality, efficiency, and value for patients. It may be how we improve, protect, and preserve our discipline as well. Our ultimate goal is to provide the people and communities we serve with the best medical care and resources we can create. We should neither toss our history and traditions aside lightly nor should we be slaves to them. This time, as all others, is a good time to consider whether we can do better.

REFERENCES

1. Polavarapu HV, Kulaylat AN, Sun S, et al. 100 years of surgical education: the past, present, and future. Bull Am Coll Surg 2013;99(7):22–7.
2. Grillo HC, Edward D. Churchill and the "rectangular" surgical residency. Surgery 2004;136:947–52.
3. Churchill ED. Personal and biographical memoirs. Taped interviews by S. Benison. Boston: Countway Library of Medicine; p. 17–25.
4. Pelligrini CA. Surgical education in the United States. Navigating the white waters. Ann Surg 2006;244(3):335–42.
5. Committee on the Governance and Financing of Graduate Medical Education, Board on Health Care Services, Institute of Medicine, et al, editors. Graduate medical education that meets the nation's health needs. Washington, DC: National Academies Press (US); 2014. 3, GME Financing. Available at: http://www.ncbi.nlm.nih.gov/books/NBK248024/.
6. CMS health care expenditures. Available at: https://www.cms.gov/Research-Statistics-Data-and-Systems/Statistics-Trends-and-Reports/NationalHealthExpend Data/downloads/highlights.pdf. Accessed September 7, 2015.
7. Meara MP, Schlitzkus LL, Witherington M, et al. Surgical resident education: what is the department's price for commitment? J Surg Educ 2010;67(6):427–31.
8. American Board of Surgery. Booklet of Information 2014-2015. Philadelphia. Available at: http://www.absurgery.org/xfer/BookletofInfo-Surgery.pdf.

Fellowship Training
Need and Contributions

Brandon T. Grover, DO*, Shanu N. Kothari, MD

KEYWORDS

- Surgical education • Fellowship • Surgical specialties • Surgical residency
- Advanced laparoscopy • Board certification

KEY POINTS

- Most graduating surgery residents pursue fellowship training.
- The current status of residency training and multiple societal changes have contributed to the increased reliance on fellowship training.
- Surgery fellowships provide the opportunity to master surgical skills, gain confidence and progressive autonomy, and receive further mentorship before entering independent practice.
- Surgical education is a dynamic process that will continue to evolve as we face the challenges ahead. Despite these challenges, North American residencies and fellowships are among the best in the world.

HISTORICAL REVIEW

Eighty percent of graduating residents now apply for fellowship training.[1] In an effort to understand this phenomenon, it is beneficial to review the history and evolution of surgical education and subspecialization.

Dr William Halsted is credited with being the father of current surgical education. In 1890 he became the first chief in the department of surgery at Johns Hopkins University and around that time established the first formal general surgery residency. Halsted based his residency program on an apprenticeship model with hospital-based training. The internship had no established length of time; rather, advancement was granted when he decided the trainee was ready to progress. This internship was typically followed by 8 years of additional training as a "house surgeon."[2] Trainees typically lived in the hospital; thus, the term *residency* came into use. The system

There are no conflicts of interest to disclose.
Department of General and Vascular Surgery, Gundersen Health System, 1900 South Avenue, C05-001, La Crosse, WI 54601, USA
* Corresponding author.
E-mail address: btgrover@gundersenhealth.org

Halsted established was pyramidal in structure, that is, more residents began training than were allowed to finish. Dr Halsted is credited with training some of the key educators of surgical subspecialization, including Harvey Cushing and Walter Dandy in neurosurgery, Samuel Crowe in otolaryngology, and Hugh Young in urology.[3,4]

In the early 1920s, medical and surgical care grew increasingly complex, and participation in internships in the United States became more common. By the 1930s, the American College of Surgeons (ACS) was pressing for better surgical training. At this time, a Committee on Graduate Training in Surgery was created. The committee determined that the best approach to surgical training was through general surgery residency. The committee also established minimum standards of education in the understanding of surgical anatomy, physiology, and pathology.[5] Around the same time, multiple certifying boards in subspecialties of surgery were established, including the American Board of Surgery (ABS) (**Table 1**).[6]

In the 1940s, Dr Edward Churchill at Massachusetts General Hospital advocated for a change from the pyramidal structure of training to a rectangular model in which all residents who started training would have an opportunity to finish, so long as they showed satisfactory progress.[2,7] He thought that general surgical training could be accomplished with a 5-year residency.[6] It was not until the 1980s that the Residency Review Committee (RRC), an arm of the Accreditation Council on Graduate Medical Education (ACGME), mandated that programs shift from the pyramidal to the rectangular structure.[8]

Table 1
Timeline of American board certification of surgical specialties and subspecialties

Specialty Board	Year
American Board of Ophthalmology	1917
American Board of Otolaryngology	1924
American Board of Obstetrics and Gynecology	1930
American Board of Orthopedic Surgery	1934
American Board of Colon and Rectal Surgery	1935
American Board of Urology	1935
American Board of Anesthesiology	1937
American Board of Plastic Surgery	1937
ABS	1937
American Board of Neurologic Surgery	1940
ABTS	1948
ABS, Pediatric Surgery	1973
ABS, Vascular Surgery	1982
ABS, Surgical Critical Care	1986
ABS, Surgery of the Hand	1989
ABTS, Congenital Heart Surgery	2006
ABS, Hospice and Palliative Medicine	2008
ABS, Complex General Surgical Oncology	2012

Abbreviations: ABS, American Board of Surgery; ABTS, American Board of Thoracic Surgery.
Adapted from Bruns SD, Davis BR, Demirjian AN, et al; Society for Surgery of Alimentary Tract Resident Education Committee. The subspecialization of surgery: a paradigm shift. J Gastrointest Surg 2014;18:1526.

The drive for surgical subspecialization became more profound during World War II. Physicians who had subspecialized training were given higher military rank, increased pay, and better assignments.[2]

In the 1970s and 1980s, competition increased between general surgery specialties and subspecialized surgical groups. The ABS established board certification in multiple subspecialties, including pediatric surgery, vascular surgery, critical care, and hand surgery. The establishment of these subspecialties laid the groundwork for the current state of fellowship training (**Table 2**).

FACTORS CONTRIBUTING TO THE NEED FOR FELLOWSHIP TRAINING

Multiple factors over several decades have led to our current state of surgical education and reliance on fellowship training. Some of these are attributable to influences outside of training, and others are directly related to changes in surgical residency training. Regardless of these influences, many choose fellowship training in order to focus their clinical practice and to become known as experts in their particular subspecialty of surgery.

Among the external forces that have propelled us toward an increased reliance on fellowships for surgical training are significant advances in surgical technology. Along with these advances comes the requirement that surgeons learn entirely new sets of skills. For example, in vascular surgery it is now the standard of care to treat many conditions with endovascular or microvascular techniques. Rather than performing

Table 2
Current status of surgical specialties and subspecialties in the United States

Discipline	Certifying Body	Board Certificate	ACGME-Regulated Residency/Fellowship
General surgery	ABS	Yes	Yes
Vascular surgery	Vascular Surgery Board of the ABS	Yes	Yes
Pediatric surgery	Pediatric Surgery Board of the ABS	Yes	Yes
Surgical critical care	Surgical Critical Care Board of the ABS	Yes	Yes
Thoracic surgery	American Board of Thoracic Surgery	Yes	Yes
Colorectal surgery	American Board of Colon and Rectal Surgery	Yes	Yes
Plastic surgery	American Board of Plastic Surgery	Yes	Yes
Advanced gastrointestinal surgery	The Fellowship Council	No	No
Surgical oncology	None	No	No
Transplant surgery	None	No	No
Breast surgery	None	No	No
Endocrine surgery	None	No	No
Acute care surgery	None	No	No

Adapted from Bell RH Jr. Graduate education in general surgery and its related specialties and subspecialties in the United States. World J Surg 2008;32:2182.

surgery directly on affected vessels through larger open incisions, many vascular disease processes can be treated through arterial or venous punctures and the utilization of specialized wires, catheters, and stents. These minimally invasive vascular techniques benefit patients by decreasing morbidity and length of hospital stay.[9] Despite these technological advances and the additional training their use requires, vascular surgeons must still be trained in traditional open techniques because not all disease processes are amenable to the minimally invasive options.

Advances in energy-based sources and endomechanical (ie, stapling) devices have profoundly affected the general and thoracic surgeon. These devices and associated technologies have reshaped the landscape of surgical care. The introduction of laparoscopic/thoracoscopic surgery demands that trainees obtain a new skill set during their years of residency training. The robot has now obtained a firm footing in surgical subspecialties, such as gynecology and urology, and is breaching into the realms of colorectal and general surgery practices as well.

Public perception that better care can be provided by specialists, such as those with fellowship training, has also made subspecialization more attractive. Advertising and market forces attempt to draw patients to physicians who have subspecialty training. There have been attempts to regionalize complex surgical cases, bringing patients to centers with high volumes and fellowship-trained specialists.[8,10]

Societal changes over the last several decades have also affected surgical education. Historically it was thought acceptable to have residents see one, do one, teach one. As residents achieved seniority in their training programs, they became accustomed to operating independently.[8] This resident autonomy has been greatly diminished by Medicare regulations that require direct attending supervision and by changes in the legal climate. For all its shortcomings, the system of the past provided a framework for confidence as new surgeons completed residency and entered practice.

Expansion of surgical knowledge over the past several decades requires that trainees gain command of a far greater body of knowledge than in the past. There has also been a shift in how disease processes are treated. Conditions that, in the past, frequently required surgery, such as peptic ulcer disease, common bile duct pathology, certain traumatic injuries, and portal hypertension, are now rarely treated with surgical interventions.

Limitations placed on resident work hours directly and greatly affect current residency training. The infamous death of Libby Zion in 1984 prompted the creation of The Bell Commission in the State of New York. The Commission concluded that resident fatigue, lack of resident supervision, and unfamiliarity with the patient's complex condition led to her death. In 1989, these findings led to the creation of New York State laws that limited resident work hours to a maximum of 80 hours per week, of which no more than 24 hours could be worked consecutively. In 2003, the ACGME mandated that similar guidelines be instituted in all residency programs throughout the Unites States. This decision reduced the hours spent in surgical training by 20% over 5 years—the equivalent of a full year of hands-on surgical education.[8]

In 2011, additional work-hour restrictions and supervision regulations were placed on interns. These restrictions limited first-year trainees to no more than 16 hours of consecutive work, no at-home call responsibilities, and no in-house responsibilities without a more senior resident or attending being physically present. It also mandated at least 8 hours of off-duty time between scheduled duty periods, with a recommendation for 10 hours off.

The goals of duty-hour restrictions were to improve patient safety, resident education, and overall resident well-being. Multiple studies have attempted to quantify the impact of the duty-hour restrictions on patient safety and surgical education, with mixed results. Some studies show no change in patient safety, and others show a deleterious effect.[11,12] A recent study on the impact of the 2011 duty-hour changes on patient safety showed no difference in mortality rates, serious complications, or readmissions when compared with those of the 3 years preceding these changes.[13] In a systematic review of the literature, Ahmed and colleagues[12] evaluated publications about the impact of duty-hour restrictions on patient safety and resident education. They reviewed more than 700 published articles, of which 135 met inclusion criteria. Of the included articles, 57 were considered to be of moderate or high quality. Findings from their review show no improvement in patient safety and, in fact, a detrimental effect in higher-acuity patients. Furthermore, nearly 90% of publications reported neither improvement nor worsening of resident education. General surgery oral examination board failure rates have climbed by 44% since implementation of duty-hour restrictions.[1] Nine of the 57 studies deemed to be of moderate or high quality evaluated resident well-being. More than 70% of respondents reported improvement in quality of life with the initial duty-hour changes made in 2003, but further enhancement was not observed with the additional changes made in 2011. Results of the studies using validated measures showed no change in resident fatigue, wellness, or burnout.[12]

Whether limitations in resident duty hours have positive or negative effects is not the intended point of this discussion; rather, the point is that these changes have altered surgical education and have been a major factor in the current need for fellowship training. It is the authors' belief that many of these restrictions will continue to remain in force for the foreseeable future, thus necessitating a change in how surgical education is implemented. Opinions about what the future landscape of residency training should look like are many and varied. Some argue that we should *fix the five*. That is, we should change how we educate and become more efficient with the time we are allotted.[1,14,15] Others suggest the establishment of core general surgery training for 3 to 4 years, followed by subspecialized training for an additional 1 to 3 years.[14] This early track approach has the theoretic advantage of reserving specific cases for those who plan to do them for the rest of their career rather than distributing these cases among all residents, some of whom have no intention of performing the case in their clinical practice. One key disadvantage of this approach is the need to conduct an additional match following the initial phase of training. This approach also raises the dilemma of how residents who complete only the initial phase of training and do not go on to finish the remaining subspecialty years would fit into the profession.

Not only have duty hour changes affected residency training but the operative experience has also shifted. As mentioned previously, more diseases and conditions are treated nonoperatively than in the past. Additionally, there has been a shift from open vascular cases to endovascular techniques and a decrease in open abdominal surgery due to the explosion of laparoscopic techniques. In several of the defined categories of training, the volume of cases with which residents graduate is lower than what is deemed necessary to provide confidence in independent practice.[14,16–18]

The aggregate of these and many other factors have influenced surgical education, thus creating an environment in which fellowship and surgical subspecialized training is quickly becoming the expected pathway for most graduating surgery residents.

FELLOWSHIP TRAINING, THEN AND NOW

The practice of the general surgeon managing a broad array of diseases ranging from thoracic, vascular, alimentary tract (foregut, midgut, and hindgut), solid organ, head and neck, and skin and soft-tissue diseases has significantly shifted over the past 30 years. These diseases remain core components of resident education, but fellowship training has profoundly altered who manages them.

In the United States, more than 20 specialty fellowships of surgery are recognized, not including subspecialties of surgery, such as orthopedics, neurosurgery, urology, ophthalmology, and otolaryngology (**Fig. 1**). Traditionally, these subspecialties required 1 to 2 years of general surgery training as a prerequisite to the specialty education.[19] Some of these programs have reevaluated the need for more time in subspecialty training and have eliminated or decreased the number of years spent in general surgery. The first to do away with general surgery training was ophthalmology.[20] Neurosurgery and orthopedic surgery have since excluded this requirement as well, and there is currently one urology program that has followed suit. The perception is that there is so much to learn within the surgical subspecialty that all of the trainees' time should be spent focused on the knowledge they will need in their future practice.[19]

The first ABS-certified fellowships in general surgery included colorectal surgery, plastic surgery, and thoracic surgery. At the inception of these fellowships, it was expected that the trainees would complete a 5-year general surgery residency, followed by fellowship training. Graduates of these fellowships were considered board-eligible in both general surgery and their respective subspecialty. It was not uncommon for a trainee to spend 7 to 8 years in residency and fellowship training combined to complete their formal educational experience in order to start their own practice in surgery. In 2003, the ABS proposed an early specialization program (ESP) authorizing vascular fellowship programs to pull residents from their general surgery training after only 4 years directly into the 2-year fellowship training, thus, decreasing the total time of training from 7 years to 6 years.[21] Early specialization has the theoretic advantage of directing surgical cases to the trainee who will need it most for future practice. More recently, medical school graduates have begun matching directly into some subspecialty surgical training programs, such as vascular, plastic, and thoracic

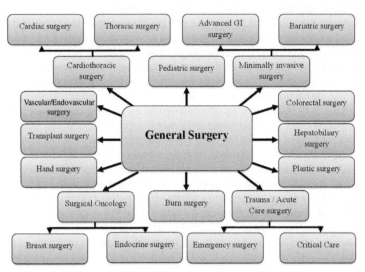

Fig. 1. The subspecialization of surgery. GI, gastrointestinal. (*Adapted from* Bruns SD, Davis BR, Demirjian AN, et al; Society for Surgery of Alimentary Tract Resident Education Committee. The subspecialization of surgery: a paradigm shift. J Gastrointest Surg 2014;18:1524; with permission.)

surgery. This training paradigm is referred to as an *integrated* pathway and consists of 3 years of general surgery training followed by 3 years of subspecialty training, all managed by the subspecialty program director.[20] Graduates from these integrated pathway programs are board eligible for their subspecialty but not necessarily for general surgery.[17]

Although pediatric surgery was authorized to participate in the ESP at the same time as vascular fellowship programs, they have elected to stay with the traditional 5 years of general surgery residency training followed by the 2-year pediatric surgery fellowship. It is theorized that the practice of pediatric surgery is similar enough to its general surgery roots that there is still a significant benefit in the knowledge and skill set attained during a general surgery residency. This training is in contrast to vascular surgery whereby there has been a major shift to endovascular treatments, drastically changing training.[20]

CURRENT STATUS OF SURGICAL FELLOWSHIPS AND SUBSPECIALTIES

The high rate of graduating residents who pursue fellowship training is not likely to decrease in the near future. There is a widespread perception that many chief residents graduate lacking the skills necessary to confidently perform some basic and many advanced laparoscopic operations.[17,18,22] Fellowships have the potential to bridge the gaps found in many residencies by providing the graduating resident with an opportunity to master surgical skills, gain confidence and progressive autonomy, and receive further mentorship. The experience also facilitates the transition from training to independent practice. Additionally, fellowship experience allows a surgeon to tailor his or her training to coincide with personal interests and future practice goals.

The number of graduating surgery residents who apply for fellowships is now more than 80%.[17,23] This number has progressively increased over the last decade and a half. In 2001, 65% of graduating surgery residents thought that they would benefit from additional training.[18] The ABS estimates that around 90% of chief residents will seek additional surgical training following graduation from general surgery residency.[24]

Some believe that the current state of fellowship training, including the rapid explosion of fellowships offered in advanced laparoscopic and gastrointestinal surgery, have placed stress on our surgical education process.[1,20,23] They contend that fellowship training has increased at the expense of residents, with the more advanced cases funneled to the fellow.

In contrast to this perception, Kothari and colleagues[25] and Hallowell and colleagues[24] independently evaluated the impact of a minimally invasive surgery (MIS) fellowship on their residency programs. Kothari and colleagues[25] looked at the number of nonbariatric advanced laparoscopic cases performed by residents both before and after the establishment of an MIS fellowship. Results from their single-institution study revealed an increase in resident experience with basic and advanced laparoscopic cases after the fellowship was created compared with before its inception: 193.3 ± 34.5 versus 140.5 ± 19.5 and 113 ± 23.5 versus 77 ± 17.8, respectively. Conclusions from their study were that a general surgery residency and an advanced laparoscopic fellowship can coexist without a detrimental effect on resident case volume. In fact, surgery residents experienced an increase in both basic and advanced laparoscopic surgery cases, while a successful fellowship was created and sustained.[24]

Hallowell and colleagues[24] performed a retrospective review of the laparoscopic operative cases for their residents and fellows over a 10-year period (2001–2011) and compared them with the national average found in the ACGME's case log system.

Their graduating chief residents performed on average 116.2 ±4.9 basic and 91.5 ±7.2 complex laparoscopic cases. During the same period, their fellows completed an average of 118 ±10.8 mostly complex laparoscopic cases as fellows and 118 ±20.9 basic and complex cases as the attending surgeon. Their resident numbers were similar to the national average and increased overall during the study period. Like Kothari and colleagues,[25] Hallowell and colleagues[24] concluded that a general surgery residency and laparoscopic fellowship can coexist. They acknowledged that a robust program was necessary in order to have adequate laparoscopic case volumes for both the resident and fellows. They believe that having the fellow enhanced the resident experience, especially when the fellow was acting as the attending during on-call responsibilities.

Not all programs have successfully sponsored concomitant laparoscopic fellowship and general surgery resident programs. Linn and colleagues,[26] from Northwestern University, described their experience of discontinuing their laparoscopic fellowship because of concerns about its adverse effect on their residency program. Although Hallowell and colleagues[24] concluded that fellowship and residency could coexist, they were obliged to decreased the number of fellows from 2 to 1 per year as bariatric case volumes declined. Therefore, each program must carefully evaluate its own circumstances and verify that it has sufficient case volume to support a fellowship program with a determined number of fellows without harming the residency training experience.

The number of advanced laparoscopic fellowship programs has increased over the past decade, from 80 in 2004 to 121 in 2015.[27] These programs and other fellowship positions are fulfilling the needs of graduating chief residents: whether to rectify a lack of experience during residency, to enhance laparoscopic skills, to become more competitive in finding a job, to focus future practice in a particular specialty, or to further their aspirations to become leaders in the field.[17,28,29]

The impact of fellowship training on future clinical practice can be difficult to quantify. In an effort to look at the benefits of laparoscopic fellowship training, researchers conducted a survey of former MIS fellows.[28] Although the response rate was low at 30%, the survey revealed that 90% of respondents thought that their fellowship was either extremely beneficial (75%) or beneficial (15%) to their career. The reasons cited for pursuing an MIS fellowship included to enhance laparoscopic skills (34%), to improve the chances of obtaining a job in a competitive market (22%), to improve the chances of becoming a future leader in the field (20%), to compensate for a lack of exposure and/or case volume during residency (19%), and to jump start a career in academics (5%).[28] Most of these MIS-trained surgeons still incorporated a broad range of laparoscopic gastrointestinal surgery into their clinical practice.

Some leaders in surgery have raised concerns that these fellowships and others that do not fall under the umbrella of board certification are unregulated and lack oversight.[1,19,20] In 2004, the American Surgical Association Blue Ribbon Committee published a report on surgical education. They described subspecialty fellowship training as, "largely unregulated, unsupervised, nonuniform, and uncertified."[30] At the time of this report, progress was already being made to correct many of the deficiencies cited. Laparoscopic fellowship programs act under the direction of the Fellowship Council (FC) established in 1997, initially known as the Minimally Invasive Surgery Fellowship Council. The initial goals of the FC were administrative in nature. They wanted to provide order to the application and match process and to properly define relationships with other organizations that were attempting to influence fellowship training. The ACS, ABS, Association of Program Directors in Surgery, and the RRC were all initially in opposition to the expansion of fellowships in MIS and advanced gastrointestinal surgery because of concerns that resident education would suffer and that the end result could lead to "franchises in gastrointestinal surgery."[23] Despite the disapproval of these influential societies, MIS fellowships have continued to expand as the perceived need for training beyond residency has skyrocketed. The FC has been instrumental in providing leadership and structure to this process.[31] The goals of the FC have shifted from where they were initially. Their main focus now is to organize and promote the development of high-quality fellowship programs.[27] The FC first provided oversight and regulation of the match process for the 2004 academic year. The FC has grown significantly since its inception and now aids in the regulation of a wide variety of fellowship programs, including advanced gastrointestinal surgery, endoscopy, MIS, bariatric/metabolic, hepatobiliary, colorectal, and thoracic surgery. More than 30% of postresidency fellowship applications are now managed by the FC.[23] The FC has been involved in the accreditation of fellowships since 2004. Individual programs are required to be in compliance with established guidelines and to submit annual reports. Every 3 years reaccreditation must occur through a formal application, and site visits are currently required every 6 years. Additionally, the FC has been instrumental in establishing a formal curriculum for each type of fellowship, which has helped to ensure uniformity in the acquisition of knowledge and surgical skills for each of the subspecialized fellowship categories.

Pursuing fellowship training is not unique to graduating general surgery residents. Ninety-five percent of responding pathology residents surveyed during their annual training examination planned to complete one or more postresidency fellowship programs. Their reasons for pursuing fellowship were similar to those given by surgery residents: to enhance skills with additional training (41%), to obtain a desired position (33%), to enhance the ability to secure employment (23%), and because a desirable job was not available immediately after residency (4%).[32]

Fellowship training provides an unparalleled opportunity to transition from formal training to independent practice. Many fellowship programs require application for hospital credentials so that fellows can take some independent calls.[28] This requirement affords fellows the autonomy that they typically did not experience during residency training and helps boost their confidence in managing emergency and acute surgical cases. Fellowship programs that have an associated surgery residency give fellows the opportunity to become the teacher. In this role, fellows have the opportunity to significantly enhance resident education.

The authors believe that MIS fellowships have been the true model for transition to practice over the past several decades. MIS fellowship training fits within the realm of general surgery; but the fellowship year provides additional mentorship and an environment capable of providing confidence and autonomy, both in and out of the operating room. Results of a survey about anticipated practice patterns after fellowship training indicated that none of the respondents planned to have a bariatric-only surgical practice.[29] Thus, most graduating MIS/bariatric fellows enter a surgery practice in which general surgery remains a significant component. MIS fellowship-trained surgeons can use the skills and knowledge attained during fellowship to educate other surgeons and, equally important, to provide expert care to surgical patients. Many of the challenges found in today's surgical education climate can be overcome by fellowship training without sacrificing the practice of general surgery.

Although the precise nature of surgical education as we move forward is uncertain, the future is bright. At no other time in history have we had the resources available that we do now. We have outstanding residencies and fellowships, state-of-the-art technology, and major advances in surgical education and simulation. Surgical education in North America continues to draw applicants from all over the globe because our training programs are widely recognized as among the best in the world.

REFERENCES

1. Lewis FR, Klingensmith ME. Issues in general surgery residency training – 2012. Ann Surg 2012;246:553–9.
2. Grillo HC. To impart this art: the development of graduate surgical education in the U.S. Surgery 1999;123:1–14.
3. Imber G. Genius on the edge: the bizarre double life of Dr. William Stewart Halsted. New York: Kaplan Publishing; 2010.
4. Harvey AM. Halsted's innovative ventures in the surgical specialties: Samuel J. Crow and the development of otolaryngology at Johns Hopkins. Johns Hopkins Med J 1977;140:101–20.
5. Ludmerer KM. Time to heal: American medical education from the turn of the century to the era of managed care. New York: Oxford University Press; 1999.
6. Bruns SD, Davis BR, Demirjian AN, et al, Society for Surgery of Alimentary Tract Resident Education Committee. The subspecialization of surgery: a paradigm shift. J Gastrointest Surg 2014;18:1523–31.
7. Grillo HC, Edward D. Churchill and the "rectangular" surgical residency. Surgery 2004;136:947–52.
8. Bell RH Jr, Banker MB, Rhodes RS, et al. Graduate medical education in surgery in the United States. Surg Clin North Am 2007;87(4):811–23.
9. Paravastu SC, Jayarajasingam R, Cottam R, et al. Endovascular repair of abdominal aortic aneurysm. Cochrane Database Syst Rev 2014;(1):CD004178.
10. Birkmeyer JD, Stukel TA, Siewers AE, et al. Surgeon volume and operative mortality in the United States. N Engl J Med 2003;349:2117–27.
11. Rajaram R, Chung JW, Jones AT, et al. Association of the 2011 ACGME resident duty hour reform with general surgery patient outcomes and with resident examination performance. JAMA 2014;312:2374–84.
12. Ahmed N, Devitt KS, Keshet I, et al. A systematic review of the effects of resident duty hour restrictions in surgery: impact on resident wellness, training, and patient outcomes. Ann Surg 2014;259:1041–53.
13. Scally CP, Ryan AM, Thumma JR, et al. Early impact of the 2011 ACGME duty hour regulations on surgical outcomes. Surgery 2015. [Epub ahead of print].
14. Cogbill TH. Surgical education and training: how are they likely to change? J Am Coll Surg 2015;220:1032–5.
15. Stain SC, Cogbill TH, Ellison EC, et al. Surgical training models: a new vision. Broad-based general surgery and rural general surgery training. Curr Probl Surg 2012;49:565–623.
16. Bell RH Jr. Why Johnny cannot operate. Surgery 2009;146:533–42.
17. Coleman JJ, Esposito TJ, Rozycki GS, et al. Early subspecialization and perceived competence in surgical training: are residents ready? J Am Coll Surg 2013;216:764–71.
18. Rattner DW, Apelgren KN, Eubanks WS. The need for training opportunities in advanced laparoscopic surgery. Surg Endosc 2001;15:1066–70.
19. Pellegrini CA, Warshaw AL, Debas HT. Residency training in surgery in the 21st century: a new paradigm. Surgery 2004;136:953–65.
20. Bell RH Jr. Graduate education in general surgery and its related specialties and subspecialties in the United States. World J Surg 2008;32:2178–84.
21. Pappas TN, Hanish SI. Don't be afraid of change: a commentary on surgical training and the American Board of Surgery. Ann Surg 2004;239:140–1.

22. Mattar SG, Alseidi AA, Jones DB, et al. General surgery residency inadequately prepares trainees for fellowship: results of a survey of fellowship program directors. Ann Surg 2013;258:440–9.
23. Fowler DL, Hogle NJ. The fellowship council: a decade of impact on surgical training. Surg Endosc 2013;27:3548–54.
24. Hallowell PT, Dahman MI, Stokes JB, et al. Minimally invasive surgery fellowship does not adversely affect general surgery resident case volume: a decade of experience. Am J Surg 2013;205:307–11.
25. Kothari SN, Cogbill TH, O'Heron CT, et al. Advanced laparoscopic fellowship and general surgery residency can coexist without detracting from surgical resident operative experience. J Surg Educ 2008;65:393–6.
26. Linn JG, Hungness ES, Clark S, et al. General surgery training without laparoscopic surgery fellows: the impact on residents and patients. Surgery 2011; 150:752–8.
27. The Fellowship Council. Available at: https://fellowshipcouncil.org/. Accessed July 1, 2015.
28. Grover BT, Kothari SN, Kallies KJ, et al. Benefits of laparoscopic fellowship training: a survey of former fellows. Surg Innov 2009;16:283–8.
29. Park A, Kavic SM, Lee TH, et al. Minimally invasive surgery: the evolution of fellowship. Surgery 2007;142:505–11.
30. Debas HT, Bass BL, Brennan MF, et al. American Surgical Association Blue Ribbon Committee report on surgical education: 2004. Ann Surg 2005;241:1–8.
31. Swanstrom LL, Park A, Arregui M, et al. Bringing order to the chaos: developing a matching process for minimally invasive and gastrointestinal postgraduate fellowships. Ann Surg 2006;243:431–5.
32. Rinder HM, Frank K, Wagner J. ASCP fellowship & job market surveys. A Report on the 2013 RISE, FISE, FISHE, NPISE, PISE, and TMISE surveys. Available at: http://www.ascp.org/PDF/Fellowship-Reports/ASCP-Fellowship-Job-Market-Surveys.pdf. Accessed July 1, 2015.

Surgical Residency Training at a University-Based Academic Medical Center

Rebecca L. Hoffman, MD[a],*, Jon B. Morris, MD[b],
Rachel R. Kelz, MD, MSCE[c]

KEYWORDS

- Surgical education • University-based • Graduate medical education
- Surgical workforce

KEY POINTS

- The tripartite mission of the university-based academic medical center defines their critical role in training surgical leaders and advancing surgery.
- The transition from an experiential model of education to an outcomes-based model has forced a critical paradigm shift in surgical education.
- The rich educational milieu of the university-based setting affords trainees a large variety of opportunities to excel in clinical care and surgical scholarship.
- An increased national focus on population and preventive health and on quality outcomes presents unique challenges to university-based departments, and by association, to the way in which residents are trained.

University-based surgical education stands at a crossroad in time. In the midst of the transition from an experiential model of education to one based on outcomes, the concepts of educational and clinical outcomes shape the way the modern generation is trained and yet, the concepts remain abstract from a practical perspective. The juxtaposition of achieving high value educational and clinical outcomes seems to be an impossible task. However, the university-based medical center, built on the principles of excellence in patient care, innovation and experimentation, and education offers

Disclosure Statement: Dr R.L. Hoffman is supported by a grant from the Measey Foundation (Grant #548018).
a Department of Surgery, Perelman School of Medicine at the University of Pennsylvania, 4 Maloney Building, 3400 Spruce Street, Philadelphia, PA 19104, USA; b General Surgery Residency Program, Department of Surgery, Perelman School of Medicine at the University of Pennsylvania, 4 Maloney Building, 3400 Spruce Street, Philadelphia, PA 19104, USA; c General Surgery Residency Program, Department of Surgery, Perelman School of Medicine at the University of Pennsylvania, 4 Silverstein Building 3400 Spruce Street, Philadelphia, PA 19104, USA
* Corresponding author.
E-mail address: Rebecca.hoffman@uphs.upenn.edu

hope that the task can be achieved and will ultimately result in a better surgeon product than was previously possible.

University-based academic institutions have long operated with the primary mission of improving health via the three pillars of clinical service, research, and education. Although providing exemplary care to patients is a common goal of all medical centers regardless of affiliation, it is the university-based medical centers' contributions to the understanding of human disease through research, dedication to technological innovation, and the education of future leaders in health care that set them apart. Ironically, these very advances in health care delivery have introduced new challenges to graduate medical education (GME).

Historically, surgical education was tied exclusively to inpatient care, because this was the epicenter of the surgical experience. The reimbursement model for training surgeons was built on this premise. This year is celebrated the 50th anniversary of the date when President Johnson signed the Medicare Act that provided hospital compensation for the direct and indirect medical expenses incurred by physicians in training.[1] The antiquated way in which surgical trainees are paid highlights how far medical education has come and how far it still needs to go to meet the needs of the modern surgical trainee.[2] Today, the nature of surgical care has changed.[3] Surgical length of stay is a fraction of what it was and two-thirds of surgical procedures are provided in the outpatient setting.[4,5] As such, surgical education has extended beyond the hospital walls despite the tethering of GME reimbursement to the hospitals.

Public perception of surgical outcomes has changed and excessive work hours and experiential training that includes practice on patients is no longer acceptable. The necessity to train residents is somewhat at odds with the commitment to provide optimal patient care.[6] Therefore, duty-hour reform and the requirements for a simulation training system to allow the acquisition of skills before patient contact has been implemented to protect the public.[7,8] Furthermore, recognition of the importance of teamwork and communication have fostered a new structure for the safe delivery of surgical care. This necessitates an expansion of surgical skills beyond technical training to adequately prepare surgeons to practice in the new world order.

Amid these paradigm shifts in the delivery of care and concomitant changes to the training environment, there is enormous pressure on the surgical workforce to generate revenue for health systems, especially in the university setting.[9] The structure of the relationship between the hospital and the university can vary significantly and often influences the surgical training environment. Large taxes placed on physician practices can shift the focus from patient care, education, and research to high-volume productivity and lead to a malalignment of incentives. Ironically, high-volume surgical practices are the cornerstone of training. Despite an outcomes-based education system, surgical education will always be centered on experience.

The real challenge for university-based academic medical centers moving forward is staying true to their tripartite mission of clinical service, research, and education. The world is more complex and these centers have to redefine themselves to meet the demands of our time. It is against this incredibly dynamic backdrop, with the university mission in mind, that we that we turn to a more thorough discussion of the state of surgical education in the university-based academic program.

PREPARING RESIDENTS TO ENTER THE SURGICAL WORKFORCE

The purpose of surgical training is to prepare physicians to care for the surgical needs of the population. To do so requires exceptional technical training in addition to teaching the skills required to foster a culture of quality and patient-centered care. Creating technically and socially competent and confident surgeons is the mission of all training programs irrespective of affiliation.

Balancing clinical demands and outcomes against the learning environment and the training needs of the surgical housestaff is a struggle for residency programs across all settings. The university-based academic programs must not only meet these needs, but also go beyond the training of expert surgeons to train physicians to become surgical leaders.[10,11] Cultivating excellence in leadership and a dedication to advancing surgery has been the educational mission of university-based academic centers since the adoption of the modern residency training structure.

The university-based programs have always strived to produce surgeons formed in their own image. Historically, this has meant training the resident to become a "triple threat": one who excelled technically; was an engaging and motivating teacher; and on top of it all, was an accomplished scientist.[12] This concept remains viable in modern times. However, rapidly advancing technology and the need for innovation has driven the expansion of the surgical scientist from the bench to a variety of additional settings. In today's surgical practice, the individual "triple threat" may excel in clinical care and teaching, and in education, basic science, quality science, health services research, the science of implementation, or a host of other areas of emerging importance in the care of the surgical patient.[12,13] Academic surgery is not an oxymoron; more opportunities for training leaders in surgery exist than ever.

An extension of the modern team-based environment, the triple threat now also exists at the department level. Individual faculty members can elect to be on tracks that maximize their job satisfaction based on their passion within surgery. Some can concentrate their efforts on clinical surgery alone, whereas others attempt the individual triple threat. Together, the collective expertise contributes to a strong department that excels in all three missions. Career tracks for academic surgeons include the busy clinical surgeon, the clinical investigator, the surgical educator, and the surgical scientist. Each has a different nonclinical focus, and different specific goals, yet all contribute to the success of surgical departments, the advancement of surgery as a discipline, and the training of future surgeons.[12]

Residents training in the university-based setting benefit from the universal interests of a diverse faculty. They learn to practice surgical skills and decision-making in innovative simulation centers. They care for a large volume of complex patients and gather substantial experience before practice. Most university-based trainees also opt for fellowship training. The combination training prepares graduates to care for general surgical patients on the transition to practice and to provide more focused subspecialty care as the graduate matures.[14]

University-based academic programs, often in urban locations, must also fulfill an obligation to train a diverse surgical workforce that can accommodate the needs of the population. Evidence that patients choose physicians of their own race, ethnicity, and gender means that recruitment of underrepresented minorities to surgical residency is important.[15,16] In addition, given the recent political and social attention surrounding lesbian, gay, bisexual, and transgender issues, training programs need to recognize that creating a diverse surgical workforce also includes attention to this other underrepresented minority.[17]

In response to duty-hour reform, university-based academic programs have had to restructure the training model. The university-based programs, often considered resource rich, house sophisticated simulation centers to permit the acquisition of clinical skills outside of the patient care arenas. Moreover, a fleet of educators across specialties enjoy teaching and self-selecting to work in a training environment provides a graduated level of responsibility. Advanced practitioner programs and ancillary support staff have expanded dramatically to reduce the amount of "service" that residents must perform to maximize the educational value of the reduced training time. And, in so doing, the program fosters an environment reliant on communication and teamwork that serves surgical trainees well throughout their professional lives.

SURGICAL SCHOLARSHIP

One of the hallmarks of the university setting is the opportunity that residents have to gain exposure to and experience in a wide range of opportunities during 1 to 3 years of dedicated research/laboratory time. In 2009, 85% of university programs had more than 5% of their residents participating in full-time research activities, compared with 34% of university-affiliated and 4% of independent academic programs.[18] At a single center, the number of residents completing greater than 1 year of research time more than doubled over the course of two decades (1990–1999, and 2000–2009).[19] This protected time is special in that it builds collegiality with faculty, allows trainees to explore their interests, develops leadership skills, and even enriches the productivity of the faculty. Prior studies have shown a strong positive correlation with research during training and the pursuit of an academic career.[20,21]

Residents spend time in the laboratory protected from major clinical duties to explore interests that advance surgical science in multiple ways. The description pays homage to a time when all surgical scholarship was in the basic sciences. More recently, a substantial portion of residents participate in translational, education, and/or quality and patient safety research. Many pursue advanced degrees (**Fig. 1**).[18] Interest in pursuing research outside of the basic sciences has been driven by several factors. Trainees have a greater interest in the public's health and well-being, consistent with a shift in generational priorities. As such, they express intellectual curiosity in new areas of health care.[22,23]

There has also been a shift in funding priorities to reflect national needs. The National Institutes of Health budget has decreased by 20% since 2004 and has had a huge impact on grant funding, especially for basic science laboratories.[24] However, monies are awarded through the Patient-Centered Outcomes Research Institute, created by the Affordable Care Act (ACA), because of the concern that traditional

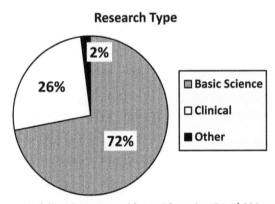

Research Type

2% / 26% / 72%

■ Basic Science
□ Clinical
■ Other

Fig. 1. Type of research fellowship pursued by residents in 131 of 239 residency programs. (*Adapted from* Robertson CM, Klingensmith ME, Coopersmith CM. Prevalence and cost of full-time research fellowships during general surgery residency. Ann Surg 2009;250(2):352; [author reply: 352]; with permission.)

medical research fails to answer questions about health outcomes that patients and clinicians wrestle with every day.[25] Also, to improve the health of communities and to improve the quality of care delivered, there has been increased access to administrative databases and the development of registries for all types of diseases. The increased use of data sources that explore patient-reported outcomes and quality metrics reflects the civic-minded values of the younger generations in the surgical workforce.[22]

Surgeons have also recognized the benefits of advanced degrees. University-based academic programs allow access to a robust body of educational opportunities. As the business of health care becomes increasingly more complex and research methodology becomes increasingly sophisticated, advanced training is useful to the future academic surgeon. Degrees in business administration (MBA), public health (MPH), health policy (MSHP), epidemiology and biostatics (MSCE), and adult education (MSEd) are just a few of the degrees available. Surgeons are increasingly taking advantage of these opportunities, rather than relying solely on observation and mentorship, to more formally develop the expertise and leadership skills necessary to make the most meaningful impact on the future of health care in this country.[26]

THE MULTIGENERATIONAL WORKFORCE

The structure and composition of the university-based academic program can influence its success. Programs must be prepared to adapt to the unique nature of the surgical workforce in the twenty-first century. Longer lifespans and career lengths mean that for the first time ever, five generations are working together and therefore learning together (**Table 1**). To further complicate the issue, contemporary trainees have quite different attitudes and expectations toward their training when compared with surgeons who trained in the pre-work-hour-reform era.[27]

Trainees of the twenty-first century belong to Generation Y, a group otherwise known as the "Millennials." Born from 1980 to 1999, they are considered an optimistic, culturally tolerant, diverse, caring group who are community-oriented and more politically engaged than previous generations. They highly value a good balance of work and home activities, tend to pursue multiple interests, and prefer immediate feedback (**Box 1**).[23] The implications of these values on surgical training and the future of the surgical workforce are profound. The nearly simultaneous launch of duty-hour reform with the entrance of the first waves of Millennials into training has not made adapting any easier. Educators have had to learn to communicate and educate in new ways and to improve educational efficiency.[22]

Surgeons have recognized the Millennials' desire for a better work-life balance, and have seen this translate into difficulties with attracting medical students into the field and into a relatively high attrition rate.[28–30] Despite duty-hour reform that limits work to 80 hours per week, attrition rates remain stable in comparison with the prereform era (0.8 vs 0.7 residents/program). Notably, residents who leave surgery continue to cite personal/lifestyle issues as the reason.[31] Proper selection of residents is of the utmost importance for the future of the surgical workforce, yet perhaps one of the most difficult tasks of a training program. There is little other than US medical licensing examination scores to provide objective data on an applicant. Most programs place the greatest weight on the interview, which is entirely subjective in nature but has the highest likelihood of revealing a student's lifestyle preferences and degree of grit, or sense of perseverance and passion.[32,33] The University of Pennsylvania has shown that it is possible to decrease attrition with an optimized selection strategy using a short prompted essay and a structured, standardized interview.[34]

Table 1
Examples of cultural and generational differences as it pertains to training and careers

Characteristics	Traditionalists	Baby Boomers	Generation X	Millennials
Years of Birth	1925–1945	1946–1964	1965–1985[a]	1978–1990[a]
Career goals	Build a legacy.	Build a stellar career.	Build a portable career.	Build a parallel career.
Balance	Support me in shifting the balance.	Help me balance everyone else and find meaning myself.	Give me balance now, not when I am 65.	Work is not everything. I need flexibility so I can balance all activities.
Rewards	The satisfaction of a job well done.	Money, title, recognition, the corner office.	Freedom is the ultimate reward.	Work that has meaning to me.
Feedback	No news is good news.	Feedback once a year, with lots of documentation.	Sorry to interrupt, but how am I doing?	Feedback whenever. I want it at the push of a button.
Training	I learned the hard way; you can too!	Train them too much and they will leave.	The more they learn, the more they stay.	Continuous learning is a way of life.

[a] There is some debate as to the date ranges that separate Generation X from Generation Y (the Millennials).

Adapted from Lancaster LC, Stillman D. When generations collide: who they are. Why they clash. How to solve the generational puzzle at work. New York: Harper Collins Publishers; 2002.

Box 1
Educational summary of Millennials

Personality

- Optimism
- Structure
- Team orientation
- Confidence bordering on entitlement

Learning Environment

- Less formal
  - Combine structured learning with group-based practical learning

Learning Style

- Prefer
  - Frequent feedback
  - Fairness
  - Recognition
  - Peer learning

Adapted from US Chamber of Comerce Foundation. The millennial generation research review. Available at: http://www.uschamberfoundation.org/millennial-generation-research-review. Accessed June 5, 2015.

University-based programs have also started to demonstrate flexibility and attention to the needs and desires of newer generations by implementing changes in departmental structure. Although departments with hierarchical models are common, they may become dated as the generations that comprise the workforce change. Economic models and family models are becoming more common as the workforce demands rewards for effort and increased flexibility.[35,36] Trainees in academic programs can see success modeled in many different ways as a manifestation of the various career/promotional tracks that are now available at many universities.[36]

The nearly simultaneous launch of duty-hour reform with the entrance of the first waves of Millennials into training has contributed to skepticism regarding the readiness of trainees for practice, and therefore the sustainability of a strong surgical workforce.[37] The different attitudes characteristic of the multigenerational surgical workforce are reflected in their perspectives on this issue of readiness as demonstrated by an American College of Surgeons survey. Whereas young surgeons endorsed preparedness for an attending role and focused on business and practice issues as barriers to autonomy in their training, older surgeons questioned preparedness, citing issues intrinsic to residency training.[38]

Because of the greatest workforce challenges that surgery faces is a shortage of generalists, training general surgeons is one obstacle that university programs, in particular, may struggle to overcome.[39] Among other reasons for specialization, residents who set their sights on a career in academic surgery see specializing as a means to achieving the kind of work-life balance that Millennials desire. Being an expert in one area tends to afford the kind of flexibility that is necessary to succeed in the academic arena. So, the university program finds itself with an educational conundrum of sorts with respect to this workforce challenge. Although supporting residents' pursuit of specialty training (when it is known that operative volume has an impact on outcomes) benefits academic surgery, it may come at the cost of perpetuating the generalist shortage. The challenge facing surgical educators on this issue is to reconcile the perspectives of multiple generations to find a common and actionable truth that ensures the sustainability of a competent, confident surgical workforce.

GLOBAL SURGERY

Another notable characteristic of this generation of surgical trainees is their commitment to public health and the global community. Medical students and residents are increasingly seeking global surgery opportunities.[40] In the last decade, the number of programs offering international electives has nearly doubled.[18] Many university-based programs are able to take advantage of their connection to the larger institution to offer these experiences. Student and institutional desires to address current real-world issues, in combination with rich resources and an extensive alumni network, make the university setting a particularly supportive environment in which to pursue international endeavors that may not exist in other types of programs.[15,41]

Two of the most common barriers to the establishment of international surgical rotations are funding and scheduling difficulties.[42] In the university setting, where departmental, hospital, and philanthropic funds may be more readily available, and where residents typically have protected research time, overcoming these barriers is more easily accomplished. Furthermore, university programs with established international rotations might enhance the training of the surgical workforce by allowing residents from other institutions to participate in their programs.

Early successes at programs, such as the University of California at San Francisco and the Alpert Medical School at Brown University, have demonstrated the impact that international experiences can have on residents and on the communities they serve.[43,44] The evidence in support of these rotations is such that the Accreditation Council for Graduate Medical Education, the Residency Review Committee, and the American Board of Surgery now allow cases performed and time spent abroad to count toward program completion.[45] Independent of case numbers, the University of Pennsylvania surgery elective in Botswana serves as an alternative experience in Systems Based Practice.[46] International rotations serve several purposes that include attracting medical students to the field, satisfying a globally conscious generation of trainees, and perhaps more importantly training a surgical workforce that is savvy in the practice of surgery in resource-poor environments.

FUNDING FOR GRADUATE MEDICAL EDUCATION

The current state of GME funding is particularly salient in the discussion of the training of the surgical workforce. There are currently 251 allopathic surgical residency programs in the United States, about half of which are university based. Funding for GME is supplied primarily by Medicare, and amounts to about $15 billion annually.[47] For the past 18 years, despite the need to close gaps in care as a result of duty-hour reform, the Balanced Budget Act has capped the number of residency slots at each program. Therefore, when it comes to funding the additional full-time equivalents, who are necessary but not funded with GME dollars, university-based academic programs may have an advantage over other types of programs. Private funding sources and endowments help to offset the costs of compliance with duty-hour reform.

Also, endowed professorships can significantly contribute to the richness of the training program by compensating faculty for time spent on educational activities. In recognition of the contributions made by teaching faculty, many universities have had the ability to and the interest in developing the clinician-educator track that provides compensation for such efforts as curricular development, didactic instruction, and educational research.[13] Many smaller independent programs rely on the volunteer efforts of their surgeons for designing and implementing an educational program that is compliant with the myriad of training requirements.

Staying true to the research mission is also not without its costs. Despite some expanded flexibility in the funding of residents by the ACA, research time, regardless of whether mandated by a program, is not covered.[48] To support resident salaries and benefits during research fellowships, it is estimated to cost $41.5 million annually.[20] Although some programs require residents to obtain external sources of funding, most programs use departmental funds to support their research residents. For residents interested in pursuing a subspecialty career, which is a significant proportion of graduates from university programs, a productive time spent doing research is viewed as necessary for obtaining a competitive postgraduate fellowship and for continuing a career in academic surgery.[6] Encouraging these academic endeavors during residency is important for the future of academic surgery.

ASSESSING THE QUALITY OF GRADUATE MEDICAL EDUCATION

GME is not exempt from the scrutiny, nor should it be exempt from the innovation that is required to reform health care in this country. A major foundation of the ACA is an emphasis on the value of care delivery as a function of decreasing costs and improving quality. Just as the quality of care delivery has been subjected to the reporting of objective measures, the demand to objectively assess the quality of GME is real. The subjective ranking of training programs based largely on peer-supplied academic reputation is no longer the sole acceptable measure of program quality in this data-driven, socially conscious era.[49]

Given the way in which surgical care is delivered in training programs (care delivered by resident teams, led by a chief resident, overseen in varying respects by an attending faculty), the methodology required to link outcomes with resident-specific patient-care activities is complex, and the resources are great.[50,51] Increased use of and access to administrative claims databases and registries have made it possible to link patient outcomes with individual surgeons and even training programs.[50,52,53] University programs are resource-rich with the kind of intellectual capital and educational monies that can help materialize the linkage between outcomes and resident practice to allow objective comment on GME quality.

BARRIERS AND CHALLENGES

The same characteristics of university academic programs that uniquely contribute to their ability to create high-quality surgical leaders also make them vulnerable in this changing health care climate. More specifically, those issues that affect the way that universities function, and by association education, are as follows[54]:

- The competitive drive to provide all services to all people, regardless of cost.
- A sense of responsibility to the public, and expectation by the public, to research and provide the latest and greatest in diagnosis and treatment.
- Reimbursement policies that are shifting, somewhat clumsily, from a high volume–high payment reward structure to a value-based reward program.
- Increased emphasis on preventive health care, and thereby a shift from individual "sickness care" to population health care.
- Increased emphasis on the delivery of high-value care via higher-quality care at a lower cost.
- Changes in reimbursement and patient referral patterns.
- Increasing pressures to generate professional fees.
- Ambiguous criteria for promotion and tenure.
- Decreased national funding and therefore increased competition for research dollars.
- Increased focus on population health and preventive care.
- Duty-hour reform.

Yet, trainee exposure to these pressures and to the innovations and adaptations that occur as a result is part of what creates the rich learning environment that is emblematic of university-based academic programs. It is this very environment that is conducive to creating new surgical leaders who are well acquainted with the issues facing the field.

SUMMARY

The first priority for university-based academic programs is to prepare trainees to meet the clinical needs of patients. Understanding the nuances of the educational mission, the type of trainee that seeks a university program, and the unique opportunities afforded to residents in a university-based academic program explains why this type of program has historically produced most leaders in surgery. University-based medical centers are well positioned to meet the challenges put before them and to continue to innovate and improve the science of surgical education to meet the evolving needs of trainees and populations that they will serve.

REFERENCES

1. Committee on Ways and Means. U.S. House of Representatives, 89th Congress, report, no. 213. Washington, DC, March 29, 1965.
2. Metzler I, Ganjawalla K, Kaups KL, et al. The critical state of graduate medical education funding. Bull Am Coll Surg 2012;97(11):9–18.
3. Lewis FR, Klingensmith ME. Issues in general surgery residency training–2012. Ann Surg 2012;256(4):553–9.
4. Hollingsworth JM, Birkmeyer JD, Ye Z, et al. Specialty-specific trends in the prevalence and distribution of outpatient surgery: implications for payment and delivery system reforms. Surg Innov 2014;21(6):560–5.
5. Weiss AJ, Barrett ML, Steiner CA. Trends and projections in inpatient hospital costs and utilization, 2003-2013. Healthcare Cost and Utilization Project, Statistical Brief #175. Rockville (MD): Agency for Healthcare Research and Quality; 2014.
6. McAlister C. Breaking the silence of the switch: increasing transparency about trainee participation in surgery. N Engl J Med 2015;372(26):2477–9.
7. ACGME program requirements for graduate medical education in general surgery. Accreditation Council for Graduate Medical Education; Section II.D.2. Effective July 1, 2014. Available at: http://www.acgme.org/acgmeweb/portals/0/pfassets/programrequirements/440_general_surgery_07012014.pdf. Accessed July 1, 2015.
8. Akhtar K, Sugand K, Wijendra A, et al. Training safer surgeons: How do patients view the role of simulation in orthopaedic training? Patient Saf Surg 2015;9:11.
9. Resnick AS, Corrigan D, Mullen JL, et al. Surgeon contribution to hospital bottom line: not all are created equal. Ann Surg 2005;242(4):530–7 [discussion: 537–9].
10. Bell RH Jr, Biester TW, Tabuenca A, et al. Operative experience of residents in US general surgery programs: a gap between expectation and experience. Ann Surg 2009;249(5):719–24.
11. Kaiser LR, Mullen JL. Surgical education in the new millennium: the university perspective. Surg Clin North Am 2004;84(6):1425–39, vii.
12. Staveley-O'Carroll K, Pan M, Meier A, et al. Developing the young academic surgeon. J Surg Res 2005;128(2):238–42.
13. Sanfey H, Gantt NL. Career development resource: academic career in surgical education. Am J Surg 2012;204(1):126–9.
14. Decker MR, Bronson NW, Greenberg CC, et al. The general surgery job market: analysis of current demand for general surgeons and their specialized skills. J Am Coll Surg 2013;217(6):1133–9.
15. Saha S, Taggart SH, Komaromy M, et al. Do patients choose physicians of their own race? Health Aff 2000;19(4):76–83.
16. Harris KM. How do patients choose physicians? Evidence from a national survey of enrollees in employment-related health plans. Health Serv Res 2003;38(2):711–32.
17. Lee KP, Kelz RR, Dube B, et al. Attitude and perceptions of the other underrepresented minority in surgery. J Surg Educ 2014;71(6):e47–52.
18. Robertson CM, Klingensmith ME, Coopersmith CM. Prevalence and cost of full-time research fellowships during general surgery residency. Ann Surg 2009;250(2):352 [author reply: 352].
19. Ellis MC, Dhungel B, Weerasinghe R, et al. Trends in research time, fellowship training, and practice patterns among general surgery graduates. J Surg Educ 2011;68(4):309–12.
20. Robertson CM, Klingensmith ME, Coopersmith CM. Prevalence and cost of full-time research fellowships during general surgery residency: a national survey. Ann Surg 2009;249(1):155–61.

21. Ko CY, Whang EE, Longmire WP Jr, et al. Improving the surgeon's participation in research: is it a problem of training or priority? J Surg Res 2000;91(1):5–8.
22. The Millennial Generation Research Review. Available at: http://www. uschamberfoundation.org/millennial-generation-research-review. Accessed June 5, 2015.
23. Vanderveen K, Bold RJ. Effect of generational composition on the surgical workforce. Arch Surg 2008;143(3):224–6.
24. Harris R, Benincasa R. U.S. science suffering from booms and busts in funding. NPR News 2014. Available at: http://www.npr.org/sections/health-shots/2014/09/09/340716091/u-s-science-suffering-from-booms-and-busts-in-funding. Accessed June 24, 2015.
25. Institute P-COR. Why PCORI was created. Available at: http://www.pcori.org/about-us/why-pcori-was-created. Accessed June 24, 2015.
26. Zheng F, Mouawad NJ, Glass NE, et al. Advanced degrees for surgeons and their impact on leadership. Bull Am Coll Surg 2012;97(8):19–23.
27. Schlitzkus LL, Schenarts KD, Schenarts PJ. Is your residency program ready for Generation Y? J Surg Educ 2010;67(2):108–11.
28. Gifford E, Galante J, Kaji AH, et al. Factors associated with general surgery residents' desire to leave residency programs: a multi-institutional study. JAMA Surg 2014;149(9):948–53.
29. Hill EJ, Bowman KA, Stalmeijer RE, et al. Can I cut it? Medical students' perceptions of surgeons and surgical careers. Am J Surg 2014;208(5):860–7.
30. Marshall DC, Salciccioli JD, Walton SJ, et al. Medical student experience in surgery influences their career choices: a systematic review of the literature. J Surg Educ 2015;72(3):438–45.
31. Leibrandt TJ, Pezzi CM, Fassler SA, et al. Has the 80-hour work week had an impact on voluntary attrition in general surgery residency programs? J Am Coll Surg 2006;202(2):340–4.
32. Makdisi G, Takeuchi T, Rodriguez J, et al. How we select our residents: a survey of selection criteria in general surgery residents. J Surg Educ 2011;68(1):67–72.
33. Salles A, Cohen GL, Mueller CM. The relationship between grit and resident well-being. Am J Surg 2014;207(2):251–4.
34. Kelz RR, Mullen JL, Kaiser LR, et al. Prevention of surgical resident attrition by a novel selection strategy. Ann Surg 2010;252(3):537–41 [discussion: 541–3].
35. Nonnemaker L, Griner PF. The effects of a changing environment on relationships between medical schools and their parent universities. Acad Med 2001;76(1):9–18.
36. Bickel J. The changing faces of promotion and tenure at U.S. medical schools. Acad Med 1991;66(5):249–56.
37. Mattar SG, Alseidi AA, Jones DB, et al. General surgery residency inadequately prepares trainees for fellowship: results of a survey of fellowship program directors. Ann Surg 2013;258(3):440–9.
38. Napolitano LM, Savarise M, Paramo JC, et al. Are general surgery residents ready to practice? A survey of the American College of Surgeons Board of Governors and Young Fellows Association. J Am Coll Surg 2014;218(5):1063–72.e31.
39. Fischer JE. The impending disappearance of the general surgeon. JAMA 2007;298(18):2191–3.
40. Powell AC, Casey K, Liewehr DJ, et al. Results of a national survey of surgical resident interest in international experience, electives, and volunteerism. J Am Coll Surg 2009;208(2):304–12.
41. Merson MH. University engagement in global health. N Engl J Med 2014;370(18):1676–8.

42. Knudson MM, Tarpley MJ, Numann PJ. Global surgery opportunities for U.S. surgical residents: an interim report. J Surg Educ 2015;72(4):e60–5.
43. Klaristenfeld DD, Chupp M, Cioffi WG, et al. An international volunteer program for general surgery residents at Brown Medical School: the Tenwek Hospital Africa experience. J Am Coll Surg 2008;207(1):125–8.
44. Ozgediz D, Wang J, Jayaraman S, et al. Surgical training and global health: initial results of a 5-year partnership with a surgical training program in a low-income country. Arch Surg 2008;143(9):860–5 [discussion: 865].
45. Accreditation Council for Graduate Medical Education. International rotation application process, Chicago. Available at: http://www.acgme.org/acgmeweb/Portals/0/PFAssets/ProgramResources/440_Surgery_International_Rotation_Application_Process.pdf. Accessed June 10, 2015.
46. The General Surgery Milestone Project. The accreditation council for graduate medical education and the American Board of Surgery. 2014. Available at: www.acgme.org/acgmeweb/portals/0/pdfs/milestones/surgerymilestones.pdf. Accessed July 6, 2015.
47. Institute of Medicine. Graduate medical education that meets the nation's health needs. Washington, DC: National Academies Press; 2014.
48. Butler PD, Chang B, Britt LD. The Affordable Care Act and academic surgery: expectations and possibilities. J Am Coll Surg 2014;218(5):1049–55.
49. Mellinger JD, Damewood R, Morris JB. Assessing the quality of graduate surgical training programs: perception vs reality. J Am Coll Surg 2015;220(5):785–9.
50. Asch DA, Nicholson S, Srinivas SK, et al. How do you deliver a good obstetrician? Outcome-based evaluation of medical education. Acad Med 2014;89(1):24–6.
51. Rajaram R, Chung JW, Jones AT, et al. Association of the 2011 ACGME resident duty hour reform with general surgery patient outcomes and with resident examination performance. JAMA 2014;312(22):2374–84.
52. Asch DA, Nicholson S, Srinivas S, et al. Evaluating obstetrical residency programs using patient outcomes. JAMA 2009;302(12):1277–83.
53. Sellers MM, Reinke CE, Kreider S, et al. American College of Surgeons NSQIP: quality in-training initiative pilot study. J Am Coll Surg 2013;217(5):827–32.
54. DiSesa VJ, Kaiser LR. What's in a name? The necessary transformation of the academic medical center in the era of population health and accountable care. Acad Med 2015;90(7):842–5.

Evolving Educational Techniques in Surgical Training

Charity H. Evans, MD, MHCM*, Kimberly D. Schenarts, PhD

KEYWORDS

- Surgical education • Training • Innovations • Educational techniques
- Medical student • Resident • Surgeon

KEY POINTS

- Surgical education has undergone a tremendous transformation since its advent in the early twentieth century, transitioning from an "apprenticeship" and "journeymanship" toward a training model based on knowledge of basic sciences, research, and graduated patient responsibility for the resident.

- Training competent and professional surgeons efficiently and effectively requires innovation and modernization of educational methods, with recognition that surgical classroom is under constant transformation, and an understanding of today's learner and learning styles.

- E-learning and the use of online curricula allows educators to overcome obstacles related to surgical education with increased accessibility of learning material, ease in updating and editing content, personalized instruction, simplicity of distribution, standardization of content, and learner accountability.

- Today's medical learner is using multiple platforms to gain information, including online surgical resources, videos, social media, and podcasts, providing surgical educators with numerous innovative avenues to promote learning.

- With the growth of technology, and the restriction of work hours in surgical education, there has been an increase in use of simulation, including virtual reality, robotics, telemedicine, and gaming. The use of simulation has shifted the learning of basic surgical skills to the laboratory, reserving limited time in the operating room for the acquisition of complex surgical skills.

INTRODUCTION

Surgical education has undergone a tremendous transformation since its advent under William S. Halsted, MD, in the early 20th century, transitioning from an "apprenticeship" and "journeymanship" toward a training model based on knowledge of

Disclosure statement: No actual or potential conflict of interest in relation to this review.
Department of Surgery, University of Nebraska Medical Center, 983280 Nebraska Medical Center, Omaha, NE 68198-3280, USA
* Corresponding author.
E-mail address: charity.evans@unmc.edu

basic sciences, research, and graduated patient responsibility for the resident. Training competent and professional surgeons efficiently and effectively requires innovation and modernization of educational methods, recognition that surgical classroom is under constant transformation, and an understanding of today's learner and learning styles. To understand today's educational climate, one must first examine the history of surgical education.

HISTORY

Study the past if you would define the future.[1]
— *Confucius*

In the early twentieth century, William Welch, the founding dean at Johns Hopkins; William Osler, Hopkins' first chief of medicine; Frederick Gates, a Baptist minister and trusted adviser to John D. Rockefeller; and Abraham Flexner, a former high school teacher, gathered as the "Hopkins Circle" and forever altered the course of medical education in the United States by advancing the science-based foundation of medical training. Flexner was invited to survey the quality of medical schools throughout America and Canada and provide suggestions for their improvement. Specifically, his assignment was to "sweep clean the medical system of substandard medical schools that were flooding the nation with poorly trained physicians."[2] Flexner's 1910 report on the state of medical education was historic, not only for its comprehensive review of all 155 medical and osteopathic institutions in the United States and Canada but because of its impact on the manner in which medicine was taught. Flexner's report is often credited with having laid the groundwork for modern medical education. Huge financial bequeaths were made by the Rockefeller and Carnegie Foundations, which in turn affected the fashion in which medical faculty would live their lives in academic medicine. Medical professors were to be freed from patient care responsibilities so as to dedicate their lives to teaching and research. At the time, most hospitals reluctantly tolerated medical student teaching. Students could receive good training in physical diagnosis and the use of certain medical instruments, but they were rarely permitted to have responsible contact with patients. Acting on his firm belief in the value of learning from patients, Sir William Osler, MD, in 1893, introduced the concept of clinical clerkships, and incorporated bedside rounds into student classes at Johns Hopkins University and, thus, the first true teaching hospital.

Paralleling medical education, surgical education has also undergone significant changes since its origin. Up until the nineteenth century, surgeons learned their craft through "apprenticeship,"[3] similar to the modern day surgical residency, followed by a "journeysmanship,"[4] similar to the modern day surgical fellowship. The typical surgical apprenticeship in the mid-sixteenth century started at approximately age 12 and lasted 5 to 7 years.[5] The young surgeon-to-be learned the craft through direct observation, then imitating the actions of a skilled mentor, both in the operating room and at bedside, providing history to the popular saying: "See One, Do One, Teach One." The masters taught with the same principle as the popular saying, they taught what they themselves had "seen" and "done." Without structure for what should be taught, guiding principles for training, or investigative inquiry for new methods or practices, medical education reached an unfortunate standstill by the late nineteenth century. The beginning of the twentieth century marked the first major shift from "apprenticeship" training to surgery residency as we know it today. The surgical training model used to train residents in the United States for the past century is, in part, due to the principles laid forth by William S. Halsted, MD, FACS.[6] The Halstedian training model was built on the triad of surgical education: knowledge of basic sciences, research, and graduated patient responsibility for the resident.

The American College of Surgeons (ACS) was formed in 1913, and has remained a strong advocate and leader in surgical education since its inception. In 1939, the ACS published the Fundamental Requirements for Graduate Training in Surgery, the first to offer criteria for hospitals that trained surgical residents, along with guidelines for achieving training criteria.[7] From 1920 to 1940, numerous medical specialty boards followed suit, and in 1928, the American Medical Association published the "Essentials of Approved Residencies and Fellowships."[8] When Medicare was approved in 1965, the medical education community realized that multiple Resident Review Committees, each with its own practices, policies, and standards, was not a coordinated standard and required focused oversight. In 1981, the Accreditation Council for Graduate Medical Education (ACGME) was born. In the years since its inception, the ACGME has strived to ensure baseline qualities in medical education through implementation of several initiatives, including the Outcomes Project in 1999, Duty-Hour Restrictions in 2003, the Next Accreditation System in 2013, and the current Milestones Project,[9] which have dramatically changed the landscape of surgical education. As governing bodies and individual training programs attempt to adapt to today's environment, we have seen an emergence of evolving educational techniques in surgical education. Just as Flexner and Halsted asked, we continue to question: How can we improve surgical education? How do we train competent and professional surgeons more efficiently and effectively? How can we reorganize surgical education to train physicians able to achieve better surgical outcomes?

CATALYST FOR CHANGE

If you aren't in over your head, how do you know how tall you are?[10]
—T.S. Eliot

Several factors served as the catalyst for change in the structure of medical and surgical education. To answer the question of how we can improve surgical education, one must first examine the shifting medical environment in which we practice today, and how the medical learner has changed from Generation X to Generation Y.

Shifting Medical Environment

In 1980, the average length of stay at teaching hospital was 7.3 days, compared with 4.5 days in 2012.[11] This change reflects technologic advances in medical care, such as improved therapeutic agents, growing use the electronic medical record (EMR), minimally invasive surgery (MIS), and efforts by the health care system to reduce hospital costs. Shorter hospital stays have changed medical education by forcing medical schools to educate in an atmosphere in which time is of the essence. As a result, students have gone from being active learners to passive observers. Furthermore, in today's clinical environment, patients are admitted with the diagnoses known and treatment plans already determined. A student on the surgery clerkship can certainly learn the technical aspects of an operation, but recognizing the symptoms of a disease process, appropriate diagnostic tests, and interpretation of those tests remains crucial to students' acquisition of clinical decision-making. Patients are frequently discharged before the effects of therapy can be observed, thus circumventing students' opportunity to follow the course of a disease and its treatment. Last, faculty are under intense pressure to be clinically productive. This pressure has resulted in many faculty having little time to teach, advise, conduct research, or serve as mentors.[12]

A Different Medical Learner

Today's medical students and surgical residents were born into the Millennial generation. The Millennial generation, or Generation Y, includes individuals born from 1982 to 2004, although precise dates vary between demographers.[13,14] Although one cannot stereotype an entire generation, the Millennials are perhaps the most studied, such that their differing traits and characteristics from Generation X become quite apparent (**Table 1**). The Millennial generation not only differs from Generation X in characteristics, but also in learning style (**Table 2**). Engels and de Gara[15] found that this generation of medical students learns by assimilation, compared with the converging style of general surgery residents and faculty. To train these learners effectively and efficiently, one must consider not only what is being taught, but how it is taught.

Millennials are "digital natives," a term coined by author Marc Prensky[16] in 2001 to describe today's students who are all "native speakers" of the digital language of the Internet, computers, and video games. Prensky[16] states that "the arrival and rapid dissemination of digital technology in the last decade of the 20th century" has changed the way "digital natives" think and process new information, making it difficult for them to excel in classrooms using outdated teaching methods commonly used in medical education today. How does this effect surgical education? Of US general surgeons currently in practice, 78% are older than 40.[17] Most surgical educators are "digital immigrants," or individuals born before the widespread adoption of digital technology, and therefore are forced to adopt the technology to survive in today's environment.[16] According to Prensky,[16] as "digital immigrants" learn to adapt in the new digital technology, they always retain certain old habits, such as reading the manual instead of assuming the program will teach us to use it or printing out e-mails to read them. Essentially, "digital immigrants" are learning a new language every day. A language learned later in life uses a different part of the brain than one learned as a primary language. Literally, "digital natives" think differently from "digital immigrants."

Table 1
Comparison of traits and characteristics of Generation X and Generation Y

Generation X	Generation Y
Year of birth: 1965–1979	Year of birth: 1982–2004
Age in 2015: 36–50	Age in 2015:11–33
Accept diversity	Celebrate diversity
Pragmatic/practical	Optimistic/realistic
Self-reliant	Self-inventive
Rejects rules	Rewrites rules
Mistrusts institutions	Irrelevance of institutions
Personal computer	Smart phones and Internet
Digital immigrant	Digital native
Uses technology	Assumes technology
Convergent learner	Assimilative learner
Multitasks	Multitasks fast
Latch-key kids	Helicopter parents

Data from U.S. Chamber of Commerce Foundation. The millennial generation research review. Available at: http://www.uschamberfoundation.org/millennial-generation-research-review. Accessed June 16, 2015.

Table 2
Comparison of traditional and evolving educational techniques

Traditional Educational Techniques	Evolving Educational Techniques
Teacher-led, memory-focused	Student-centered, performance-focused
Knowledge bestowed from authoritative source	Learner-constructed knowledge from multiple sources and experiences
Isolated work on prepared exercises	Collaborative work on real-world projects
Predetermined progression	Flexible progression
One path	Multiple paths
Single-sense stimulation, limited media	Multisensory stimulation, media-rich
Taught to one learning style	Accommodate multiple learning styles
Mastery of fixed content and specified processes	Student defines, designs, and manages project
Competence defined by facts and literal thinking	Creative thinking for innovation and original solutions
In class expertise, content, and activities	Global expertise, information, and learning experiences
Written communication and information	Digital information and communication systems
Primary focus on school and local community	International focus with digital global citizenship
Outcome-based assessment	Competency based assessment

Data from Nicholas A. Preferred learning methods of the Millennial Generation. Faculty and Staff – Articles & Papers. 2008; Paper 18.

EVOLVING TECHNIQUES IN SURGICAL EDUCATION

We need to prepare students for their futures, not our past.[18]
—*Ian Jukes*

The role of the teacher in surgical education is quickly changing. As new technologies are developed, such as online learning portals, social media outlets, and virtual reality, the surgical educator is challenged to adapt educational techniques to meet the needs of the twenty-first century medical learner.

Defining E-learning

Traditional teacher-centered didactic teaching is yielding way to a learner-centered approach in online Web-based arena. The term "e-learning" refers to the delivery of learning, training, or education programs by electronic means.[19] E-learning overcomes several educational obstacles and, therefore, is gaining popularity in surgical education. Delivery is the most commonly cited advantage of E-learning, as online curricula facilitates increased accessibility of learning material, ease in updating and editing content, personalized instruction, simplicity of distribution, standardization of content, and learner accountability.[19,20] E-learning also can potentially improve the efficiency and effectiveness of surgical education. The software used to create e-learning modules, such as Articulate, Camtasia, and Elucidat, allow educators to create a learning platform based on adult learning theory; that is, encourage the learner to relate new learning to past experiences by linking learning to specific needs, then create practical application.[21] Engaging the learner in the online environment and promoting interactivity with the material stimulates efficiency, motivation to learn, and cognitive effectiveness. Evidence suggests that e-learning is a more effective method of teaching because learners gain knowledge and skills faster than through traditional teacher-focused methods, leading to improved motivation and performance.[22] However, for e-learning to be successful, several elements must exist: content management, course design, learning objectives and measurable outcomes, and communication (**Table 3**).

Web-based tools offer several advantages over in-person/printed educational tools: few physical or time-based barriers, searchable content, and interactivity. Furthermore, students can view the material at their own pace, and review material as needed, which is not possible in a live lecture. In the current training climate, in which surgeons are expected to reach proficiency despite a decrease in work hours, e-learning can make educational time more efficient. For example, Gonzalez and colleagues[23] restructured the neurosurgical teaching program at their institution by providing trainees with tablet devices as an educational resource. The investigators report a subsequent significant improvement in examination scores: 92% of trainees attributed increased time spent studying outside of hospital to the provision of tablets, and 67% used these devices as the primary means of accessing educational resources.

Flipped Versus Blended Classroom Versus Massive Open Online Courses

If a child can't learn the way we teach, maybe we should teach the way they learn.[24]

—*Ignacio Estrada*

The advent of e-learning has introduced several new terms used to describe the use of online curricula in the classroom, including the "flipped classroom," "blended classroom," and the Massive Open Online Course. The "flipped classroom" is a concept first presented by J. Wesley Baker[25] in 2000 in "The "Classroom Flip: Using Web

Table 3 Necessary elements of e-learning	
Necessary Elements in E-Learning	**Description**
Content management	Storing, indexing, and cataloging of learning materials necessary to make content available to learners
Course design	Synchronous: real-time, instructor-led e-learning, where all learners receive information simultaneously and communicate directly with one another Asynchronous: transmission and receipt of information do not occur simultaneously, learners are responsible for pacing their own self-instruction and learning
Learning objectives and measurable outcomes	Description of what the learner should know or be able to do at the end of course, serves as basis for the larger educational materials
Teacher/student communication	Face-to-face ± online social media
Multimedia	Animations, videos, audio, print
Engagements	Opportunities for the learner to interact with the material
Assessment	Formative vs summative

Course Management Tools to Become the Guide by the Side," and by Lage and colleagues[26] in their article "Inverting the Classroom: A Gateway to Creating an Inclusive Learning Environment." In this model, what is traditionally done in class (teacher-led lecture with students listening and taking notes) is done before class, and what was traditionally homework (problems solved using information from lecture) is done in the scheduled class.[27] This model flips the traditional roles of the teacher and student, leading to the ability to cover more material, accommodation of students with different learning styles, better engagement of students with collaborative exercises, and improved assessment of understanding.

The "blended classroom" first appeared in a press release in 1999 by the Interactive Learning Centers.[28] The blended learning model allows the student to learn, at least in part, through delivery of content and instruction online, such that the student has control over time, place, path, or pace.[29] Advocates of blended learning state that incorporating the "asynchronous Internet communication technology" into higher education serves to "facilitate a simultaneous independent and collaborative learning experience"[30] and this mix of independence and collaboration leads to student satisfaction and learning success.

A Massive Open Online Course, or MOOC, is an online course aimed at unlimited participation and open access via the Internet. The MOOC was first introduced in 2008, and by 2012, emerged as a popular mode of learning.[31,32] The MOOC is a type of distance learning that incorporates traditional course materials, such as readings, problem sets, and videos with an interactive user format to support interface between learners and teachers. According to the New York Times, 2012 became the "year of the MOOC," as several online providers, associated with top academic universities, emerged.[31,33] MOOCs carry great potential in surgical education, as the learning material can reach learners regardless of time or distance, and can be used for new material, certification, or maintenance of certification. In a 2014 review, the investigators identified 98 free health and medicine-related MOOCs, of which 90 were offered by major universities. The duration of MOOCs varied from 3 to 20 weeks, with an average of 6.7 weeks. The MOOCs required an average of 4.2 hours per week of participant work, and verified certificates were offered by 14, with another 3 offering professional recognition.[34]

It is important to note that these types of online curricula are not simply the opportunity to access online lectures. The Millennial learner prefers teamwork and interactive learning by engaging with the materials, faculty, and colleagues.[35] Furthermore, online learning material works best when it addresses lower-order cognitive skills, including knowledge and comprehension. Higher-order skills, such as application and analysis, are best taught face-to-face, with faculty supervision and input.[36] Millennial learners want to have a close relationship with authority figures, similar to the relationship they grew accustomed to with their "helicopter" parents.[37] The term "helicopter" parents first appeared as a metaphor in 1969, and refers to the parent who pays extremely close attention to a child's experiences and problems, particularly in education.[38] Millennial learners also want to feel that their supervisors care about them personally, and prefer to work with superiors who are approachable, supportive, good communicators, and good motivators. This brings new function to the role of teacher. In the Halstedian era, learners were taught to think critically through "pimping," where the medical trainee was asked a series of questions designed to test the boundaries of known knowledge. However, in the current environment, there is concern about both the term "pimping" and its purpose. Kost and Chen have suggested that educators focus on questioning that "is more learner centered; aids in the acquisition of knowledge and skills; performs helpful formative and summative assessments of the leaner; and improves community in the clinical learning environment."[38] This shift from "pimping" to learner-centered dialogue can be challenging for surgical educators; however, it better meets the educational needs of today's learner.

Online Surgical Resources

Online learning is not the next big thing, it is the now big thing.[39]

—*Donna J. Abernathy*

The growth in online surgical resources speaks to the popularity of e-learning in surgical education. The Surgical Council on Resident Education (SCORE) initiative was created in 2004 to "provide residents with high-quality educational materials and a structured program for self-learning in all areas of general surgery."[40] By 2014, approximately 200 programs subscribed to the SCORE Web portal. Early data suggest that SCORE improves the education of surgical residents. Klingensmith and colleagues[41] found considerable improvement in mean qualifying exam scaled scores for residents in programs that subscribed to the Web portal.

The Web Initiative for Surgical Education of Medical Doctors (WISE-MD) is a series of Web-based modules built on the theoretic framework laid out by Dr Richard E. Mayer, who proposed that improved learning occurs when animation and narration occur simultaneously, especially if this process activates prior knowledge.[42,43] WISE-MD started in 2003 with the Computer-assisted Learning in Pediatrics Program (CLIPP) cases based on the national pediatric medical student curriculum. In 2006, the nonprofit MedU was founded to sustain CLIPP. In 2009, the WISE-MD modules for surgical education, developed by the Department of Surgery and the Division of Educational Informatics at NYU in collaboration with the Association for Surgical Education, was integrated into MedU.[44] In 2013, 99 medical schools in the United States. subscribed to WISE-MD, paralleling the popularity of online surgical resources even in graduate medical education.[45]

Dr Mayer's research prompted educators to create learning environments such as WISE-MD, and may also explain the surge of surgical videos used by learners to augment their operative experience. WebSurg, the e-Surgical reference, is a "virtual surgical university, accessible from anywhere in the world through the Internet." WebSurg is available in 6 languages, and has approximately 323,000 registered users.[46] YouTube is a video-sharing Web site founded in 2005. The site allows users to upload non–peer-reviewed videos that can be viewed anywhere in the world. It is the third most popular Web site in the world, accounting for 60% of all videos watched online. Glass and colleagues[47] surveyed members of the Resident and Associate Society of the ACS concerning educational resources used, and found that 30.8% of all respondents used online videos and lectures to prepare for examinations, 34.4% for building fund of knowledge, and 22.6% for information regarding patient care. Use of online videos and lectures was higher in senior residents compared with junior residents. This percentage is even higher in medical students. In a study by Barry and colleagues,[48] 78% of second-year undergraduate medical and radiation therapy students surveyed reported using YouTube as their primary source of anatomy-related video clips.

A Podcast is a series of audio files downloaded through Web syndication or streamed online to a computer or mobile device, whereas a Vodcast is a video podcast.[49] In a study of 112 medical students, 68% reported listening to at least one podcast (average of 6) during their general surgery clerkship. When surveyed about efficacy, 84% agreed the podcasts helped them learn core topics, and more than 80% found the recordings interesting and engaging.[50] Medical students report using podcasts and vodcasts regularly to supplement their learning in novel ways, even while driving to clinic or exercising, providing educators with yet another avenue to reach learners.[51]

Social Media

With the boom of social media in the early 2000s, educators have used this technology to promote learning. Social media is defined as "a group of Internet-based applications that build on the ideological and technological foundations of Web 2.0, and allow the creation and exchange of user-generated content."[52] The most popular forms of social media used by medical students and residents include blogs, wikis, Twitter, and Facebook (**Table 4**). Cheston and colleagues[52] reported that blogs were the most commonly used social media tool (71%) by medical students, followed by wikis (21%), Twitter (14%), and Facebook (14%). When students were asked to write essays, they generally favored blogging for the purpose of reflection, but favored in-person problem-based learning over virtual collaborative learning for improvement of clinical reasoning skills. Students who actively participated in blog-based discussion forums had higher grades than those who posted less often. Social media tools also provided opportunities for more feedback on their performance.[53] Twitter has been suggested as a medium to involve students by creating a dialogue on the subject matter through retweeting key points and messages from lecture material. Twitter enables students to continue a discussion about a lecture and tie information to current events by using hashtags.[51] Social media platforms such as Facebook also provide a powerful way to integrate medical education globally. In an *New England Journal of Medicine* Facebook group, a new "image challenge" is posted each week, and Facebook users can comment and give their diagnosis.[51]

Simulation

We are what we repeatedly do. Excellence, then, is not an act but a habit.[54]

—*Aristotle*

Table 4 Forms of social media			
Platform	**Origin**	**Usage as of 2014**	**Description**
Blog	1994	207.3 million bloggers	Short for "Web log," is an online discussion or informational site published on the Web and consists of discrete entries or "posts" typically displayed in reverse chronologic order
Wiki	1994	4.9 million wiki pages	A Web site that allows collaborative editing of its content and structure of a Web site by its users. The best known example of a wiki Web site is Wikipedia (www.wikipedia.com)
Twitter	2006	236 million users	Online social networking service that enables users to send and read short 140-character messages called "tweets" (www.twitter.com)
Facebook	2004	1.23 billion users	Online social networking service that connects people with friends and others who work, study, live, and engage around them. People use Facebook to keep up with friends, to share links, to share photos and videos of themselves and their friends, and to learn more about people and organizations (www.facebook.com)

With the growth of technology, and the restriction of work hours in surgical education, we have seen an increase in use of simulation. This is likely related to how surgical residents learn the technical aspects of surgery. Surgical residents advance through the 4 stages of learning as they progress through residency: the novice, the apprentice, the journeyman, and finally, the master.[55] Knowledge and skills are developed with repetition in a number of venues: on the wards, in the classroom, and in the operating room. Time in the operating room is limited by service duties and work hours, and, therefore, is too valuable to be used for the acquisition of basic technical skills such as knot tying and suturing. In the novice and apprentice stages of learning, complex operative tasks are deconstructed into component skills, then taught individually until mastered. Virtual reality, including mechanical simulators, robotics and telesurgery, and animate models provide learners with the opportunity to acquire familiarity with instruments, improve dexterity, and gain knowledge about management, techniques, and potential complications of treating surgical conditions.

Virtual reality (VR) is an artificial environment that is created with software and presented such that the user suspends belief and accepts it as a real environment. There are 2 important components of VR in surgical education: realism and fidelity. If the environment appears realistic, the trainee's emotional and physiologic response to the simulation will have a more accurate translation into the operating room.[56] Fidelity refers to the degree with which the artificial environment looks, feels, and acts like a human patient.[57] Mechanical simulators, or boxes in which objects or organs are placed and manipulated using surgical instruments,[58] are the most primitive and the least expensive form of VR. They can define grades of difficulty and are capable of immediate performance feedback, making mechanical simulators ideal for initial acquisition of basic skills, familiarization with instruments, and basic techniques. Computer-based simulators provide an environment to apply basic skills to more complex operations. The degree of difficulty can be altered, along with modifications of the normal anatomy, forcing the learner to make intraprocedural decisions.[59] Dutta and colleagues suggested that the unmet needs in our current training environments could be addressed by VR, to include exposure to rarely encountered conditions; focus on the learning needs of trainees in a cost-effective manner outside the OR; and performance assessment that includes decision-making, leadership, communication and judgment, all of which are difficult to assess in actual patient care.[60] For VR to fill the gaps in surgical education, simulators must be realistic and, according to surgical innovators, "accurately teach the ergonomics, dexterity, steps of procedures and the more intangible visualization all at once, without risk to the patient....The ultimate goal is to have an adaptive and intelligent training and assessment system. It should not only be level-appropriate but also have the capability to change based on recognition of the user's performance and deficiencies to this point, as well as how quickly the learner has improved in the past."[57]

Robotics

Perhaps the single greatest surgical innovation of the past 3 decades is the advent of MIS. Education and proficiency in MIS requires intensive and ongoing training, as it is technically difficult given the unnatural visual and haptic perceptions. The 2-dimensional monitor alters in-depth perception and hand-eye coordination, while the laparoscopic equipment changes force feedback while manipulating tissue.[61] Computer-integrated surgery using robotics augment the surgeon's skill by providing additional information that is less available to surgeons through human senses, specifically, with endo-wrist technology, $\times 10$ magnification and 3-dimensional vision, when compared to laparoscopic surgery. With the introduction of robotic surgery, surgical educators are now challenged with how to teach, train, and credential surgeons to use this technology. Robotic simulators were created to replicate the surgery, develop the skills necessary to perform robotic procedures, and help the surgeon learn to negotiate the "human-machine" interface.[62] Robotic surgery allows the learner to practice within countless patient scenarios created by the computer, in addition to video and calculation of hand motion data. Mistakes made in simulation do not have human consequence, and actually have a positive impact on learning under proper supervision and feedback.[63] The clearest role for robotic simulation is in practicing before performing a surgery. A presurgical warm-up gives the surgeon an opportunity to prepare for the case, with the ability to use the patient's own imaging as a 3-dimensional virtual anatomic model via the simulator software.[64,65] The major barrier to robotic simulation is cost and access, with a single robot costing approximately $800,000, with a $100,000 per year running cost.[66]

Telesurgery

The robotic surgery system allows a surgeon to perform a surgical procedure at a remote site, known as telesurgery. Telesurgery is defined as "a procedure performed on an inanimate trainer, animate model, or patient in which the surgeon is not at the immediate site of the model or patient being operated on."[67] Robotic platforms were originally developed by the military to address the need to deploy robotic surgical capabilities in forward conflict arenas. The first long-distance telesurgery procedure was successfully completed in 2002. In the clinical realm, telesurgery is limited by legal barriers, as physicians cannot practice medicine across state lines without having a medical license in each state.[68,69] The benefit of telesurgery in education is in mentoring. Telementoring, or real-time interactive teaching of techniques by an expert surgeon to a student not at the same site,[67] was first reported in 1965 by Dr Michael DeBakey, who transmitted guidance on an open heart surgery from the United States over broadband satellite to surgeons in Europe.[70] Since then, a number of laparoscopic procedures have been performed by less experienced surgeons under the guidance of more experienced surgeons. Teleproctoring, or the monitoring and evaluation of surgical trainees from a distance,[67] is used for credentialing purposes and to set a standard of care and assessment for skills across hospitals.[71] Teleconferencing and teleconsulting involve more demonstration and discussion than just interaction and intervention, where live surgeries can be transmitted for guidance and review.

Animate Models

In addition to computer-created simulation, the use of cadavers allows for the realism of real tissue, without the risks associated with learning on human subjects. Kaplan and colleagues developed an emergency surgical skills laboratory (ESSL) using a non-preserved cadaver during the third-year surgery clerkship. Students in this study were able to obtain suturing proficiency as well as important technical skills in the ESSL that were previously taught in the operating room, emergency department, or wards.[72]

Gaming

The traditional medical model of "see one, do one, teach one" is no longer adequate to train physicians, because many skills cannot be developed by merely watching an expert.[73–75] Minimally invasive operations provide an additional set of challenges that are not inherent in open operations, such as decreased tactile feedback, the fulcrum effect and working in 3 dimensions while focusing on 2.[76] Video games offer visually realistic simulations that demand the same visual-motor dexterity sought in a surgical resident. Rosser demonstrated that past video game play in excess of

3 hours per week has been correlated with 37% fewer errors and 27% faster completion. In his study, current video gamers made 32% fewer errors, performed 24% faster, and scored 26% better overall than their nonplaying colleagues. He concluded that "training curricula that include video games may help thin the technical interface between surgeons and screen-mediated applications, such as laparoscopic surgery. Video games may be a practical teaching tool to help train surgeons."[75] Similar results were found in a study of veterinary medical students, where a significant positive association was detected between summary scores for video game performance and laparoscopic skills, but not between video game performance and traditional skills scores.[77] In a study comparing video games and laparoscopy simulators in the development of laparoscopic skills in surgical residents, residents were randomly assigned to 1 of 3 interventions: a traditional laparoscopic box trainer, an Xbox gaming console, or a Nintendo DS handheld gaming system. Residents assigned to the Xbox 360 spent more time each week playing their game, and had the greatest improvement of the tested peg transfer time. Residents who reported a history of playing video games (at least 5 hours per week) performed better on the initial peg transfer than residents who reported having never played video games.[76]

Surgical Improvement of Clinical Knowledge Ops (SICKO) is an educational tool that applies gamification techniques and teaches the workup and operative management of classic surgical diseases. SICKO uses an immersive, interactive, and media-rich user interface along with a point system to reward or penalize right or wrong actions, offering instant feedback. All actions, answers, and consequences, are compiled into a final end-of-game report for the learner to review. Researchers noted expert players outperformed less experienced players, suggesting that educational games may be a valid assessment of medical decision-making.[78]

CHALLENGES OF INNOVATION IN SURGICAL EDUCATION

The mother of excess is not joy but joylessness.[79]
—Friedrich Nietzsche

Technological innovations may enhance surgical education; however, they also bring new challenges. Electronic devices used to deliver e-learning also tempt the learner to multitask, such as reading several articles at once, or checking e-mail or reviewing patient's charts while studying. Millennials are reported to be superb multitaskers. However, the science tells a different story. A study examining whether texting or posting to a social network site has negative impacts on students' learning found that students who were not using their mobile phone wrote down 62% more information in their notes, took more detailed notes, were able to recall more detailed information from the lectures, and scored a full letter grade and a half higher on a multiple choice test than those students who were actively using their mobile phones.[80] Others have investigated the relationship between classroom laptop usage and course achievement. Kraushaar and Novak developed a rubric to classify programs as productive or distractive toward the student (productive programs were course-related; distractive programs included Web surfing, e-mail, or instant messaging). They found that 62% of the programs that students had open on their laptops were considered distracting. They additionally found that instant messaging was negatively correlated with quiz averages, project grades, and final examination grades.[81]

Studies on multitasking have shown greater vulnerability to interference, leading to worse performance.[82] But, is the Millennial generation really multitasking? Newer research suggests that Millennials can switch tasks so quickly that it appears they are doing the tasks simultaneously without truly multitasking.[83] The Millennial generation appears to be rewiring the brain with fast simultaneous tasking, such as playing on the computer while watching TV and reading a book. This retraining allows the brain to reduce performance deterioration of multitasking by increasing the speed of information processing by the brain, thereby allowing multiple tasks to be processed in more rapid succession.[83]

Fast simultaneous tasking appears to be the new norm, as new technologies, such as smart phones and tablet devices, continue to grow in number and popularity. In a survey of medical students, residents, and faculty members at 4 Canadian medical schools, mobile devices were commonly used to find drug information (73.5%), perform clinical calculations (57.9%), take notes (51.6%), search for journal articles (46.5%), and read journal articles (50.2%). Medical students and residents additionally used their mobile devices to find clinical practice guidelines, read point-of-care information, do clinical calculations for performing differential diagnoses, and access medical resources.[84] In a review of smart phone uses in medicine, research has demonstrated that the smartphone is improving communication on internal medicine wards, suggesting that there may be a role for better communication between doctors and nurses.[85] A systematic review of the literature by Mobasheri and colleagues[86] demonstrated the widespread potential of smartphone and tablet platforms within surgery. Preoperatively, these technologies have been used to aid surgical diagnosis, assist in operative planning, educate patients regarding scheduled operations, and decrease anxiety in pediatric surgical patients. Intraoperatively, such technology has been used for telementoring. Postoperatively, these platforms have been used to monitor and review patients remotely. In terms of operative training, tablet devices have been used as simulators and as a means of improving accessibility to educational content both at the user's convenience and at the point-of-care delivery. In contrast to previous smart phone study results, access to EMRs was one of the most frequently reported uses of the tablet computer. The investigators speculate that tablet computers are preferred over smart phones for EMR access primarily as a result of the large displays and a greater number of integrated EMR platforms.[87]

The effect of increased use of smart phones and texting in medicine has changed the way medical professionals communicate. In a study of text messaging among residents and faculty in a university general surgery residency program, most surgery residents (88%) and attendings (71%) texted residents. Fewer residents (59%) and attendings (65%) texted other faculty. Most resident-to-resident texting occurred 3 to 5 times per day (43%), whereas most attending-to-resident texts occurred 1 to 2 times per day (33%). Among those who texted, the most frequently reported purpose was patient-related care among all groups.[88] A drawback to this technology was weakened interprofessional relationships.[85]

SUMMARY

The "Hopkins Circle" gathered in the early twentieth century, likely unaware of the tremendous impact their shared thoughts and innovation would have on medical education in the United States. Flexner's report spurred changes in the medical education, while the leadership of Osler and Halsted formed surgical residency as we know it today. A common thread throughout surgical history is the desire to improve surgical education such that graduates are competent, professional, compassionate, and safe. As technology has advanced, so has the educational armamentarium available to surgical educators. Embracing both the learning styles of this generation and the evolving technological advances, such as the "flipped" and "blended" classroom, MOOCs, videos, social media, and podcasts, is not only inevitable but necessary to engage today's medical learner. Simulation, VR, robotics, telemedicine, and gaming are no longer the future of surgical education, but represent the standard by which competence will be developed and measured. If Halsted were alive today, he may not recognize the technology and methods, but he would embrace the current academic model that fosters scientific knowledge, research, and learner and patient-centered surgical education.

REFERENCES

1. Quotes about history. Goodreads Web site. Available at: http://www.goodreads.com/quotes/tag/history. Accessed June 16, 2015.
2. Duffy TP. The Flexner report—100 years later. Yale J Biol Med 2011;84(3):269–76.
3. History of apprenticeship. Washington State Department of Labor & Industries website. Available at: www.lni.wa.gov/TradesLicensing/Apprenticeship/About/History/. Accessed on June 15, 2015.
4. "Journeyman" definition. Oxford English dictionary. 2nd edition. Oxford University Press; 2009. Available at: http://www.oxforddictionaries.com/us/definition/american_english/journeyman. Accessed June 15, 2015.
5. Dobson J, Walker RM. Barbers and barber-surgeons of London: a history of the Barbers' and Barber-surgeons companies. Oxford (United Kindgom): Blackwell Scientific Publications; Worshipful Company of Barbers; 1979. p. 171.
6. Nguyen L, Brunicardi FC, Dibardino DJ, et al. Education of the modern surgical resident: novel approaches to learning in the era of the 80-hour workweek. World J Surg 2006;30:1120–7.
7. American College of Surgeons. Centennial reprint: Graduate training for general surgery and the surgical specialties. Bulletin of the American College of Surgeons website. 2013. Available at: http://bulletin.facs.org/2013/03/reprint-graduate-training/. Accessed on June 15, 2015.
8. Eisele CW. Essentials of a residency in general practice. JAMA 1957;164:384–8.
9. Milestones. Accreditation Council for Graduate Medical Education Web site. Available at: https://www.acgme.org/acgmeweb/. Accessed June 22, 2015.
10. Quotes about challenges. Goodreads Web site. Available at: http://www.goodreads.com/quotes/tag/challenges. Accessed on June 23, 2015.
11. Vital and Health Statistics: compilations of advance data from vital and health statistics. U.S. Department of Health and Human Services, Public Health Service, Centers for Disease Control, National Center for Disease Statistics; 1989. Issue 14–18.
12. Ludmerer KM. The development of American medical education from the turn of the century to the era of managed care. Clin Orthop Relat Res 2004;422:256–62.
13. DiLullo C, McGee P, Kriebel RM. Demystifying the Millennial student: a reassessment in measures of character and engagement in professional education. Anat Sci Educ 2011;4:214–26.
14. Howe N, Strauss W. Millennials rising: the next great generation. New York: Vintage Original; 2000.
15. Engels PT, de Gara C. Learning styles of medical students, general surgery residents, and general surgeons: implications for surgical education. BMC Med 2010;10:51.
16. Prensky M. Digital natives, digital immigrants. Horizon 2001;9:1–6.

17. Walker E, Poley S, Ricketts T. The aging surgeon population, vol. 5. American College of Surgeons Health Policy Research Institute; 2010. p. 1–4.
18. Daniels M. 10 Inspirational quotes for EdTech-friendly teachers. 2011. Available at: http://www.knewton.com/blog/teacher-tools/10-inspirational-quotes-for-edtech-friendly-teachers/. Accessed June 16, 2015.
19. Rosenberg M. E-learning: strategies for delivering knowledge in the digital age. New York: McGraw-Hill; 2001.
20. Wentling T, Waight C, Gallaher J, et al. E-learning: a review of literature. Knowledge and Learning Systems Group, National Center for Supercomputing Applications, University of Illinois. 2000;1–73.
21. Gibbons A, Fairweather P. Computer-based instruction. In: Tobias S, Fletcher J, editors. Training & retraining: a handbook for business, industry, government, and the military. New York: Macmillan Reference USA; 2000. p. 410–42.
22. Clark D. Psychological myths in e-learning. Med Teach 2002;24:598–604.
23. Gonzalez NR, Dusick JR, Martin NA. Effects of mobile and digital support for a structured, competency-based curriculum in neurosurgery residency education. Neurosurgery 2012;71:164–72.
24. Ignacio Estrada Quotes. Goodreads Web site. Available at: http://www.goodreads.com/quotes/750708-if-a-child-can-t-learn-the-way-we-teach-maybe. Accessed June 24, 2015.
25. Baker JW. The "Classroom Flip": Using Web Course Management Tools to Become the Guide by the Side. Selected papers from the 11th International Conference on College Teaching and Learning. Jacksonville, FL, April 9–17, 2000.
26. Lage MJ, Platt GJ, Treglia M. Inverting the classroom: a gateway to creating an inclusive learning environment. J Econ Educ 2000;31:30–43.
27. Chambers JA. Selected papers from the 11th International Conference on College Teaching and Learning. Jacksonville, FL, April 12–15, 2000.
28. Interactive Learning Centers announces name change to EPIC learning. The Free Library Web site. 2014. Available at: http://www.thefreelibrary.com/Interactive+Learning+Centers+Announces+Name+Change+to+EPIC+Learning.-a054024665. Accessed June 23, 2015.
29. Garrison DR, Kanuka H. Blended learning: Uncovering its transformative potential in higher education. Internet High Educ 2004;7:95–105.
30. Pappano L. The year of the MOOC. The New York Times 2012. Accessed June 23, 2015.
31. Lewin T. Universities abroad join partnerships on the web. New York Times 2013. Accessed June 23, 2015.
32. Smith L. 5 education providers offering MOOCs now or in the future. Education Dive website. 2012. http://www.educationdive.com/news/5-mooc-providers/44506/. Accessed June 23, 2015.
33. Liyanagunawardena TR, Williams SA. Massive open online courses on health and medicine: review. J Med Internet Res 2014;16:e191.
34. Kurup V, Hersey D. The changing landscape of anesthesia education: is flipped classroom the answer? Curr Opin Anaesthesiol 2013;26:726–31.
35. Prunuske AJ, Batzli J, Howell E, et al. Using online lectures to make time for active learning. Genetics 2012;192:67–72.
36. Epstein M, Howe P. The millennial generation: recruiting, retaining, and managing. Today's CPA 2006;24–7.
37. Ginott H. Between parent & teenager. New York: MacMillan; 1969. p. 18.
38. Kost A, Chen FM. Socrates was not a pimp: changing the paradigm of questioning in medical education. Acad Med 2015;90:20–4.

39. Online Learning. Faculty Circle for Online Teaching Web site. 2012. Available at: https://sites.temple.edu/ollteachingcircle/2012/03/08/slide-1/. Accessed June 24, 2015.

40. The SCORE portal. SCORE Web site. 2009. Available at: http://www.surgicalcore.org/public/about. Accessed June 22, 2015.

41. Klingensmith ME, Jones AT, Smiley W, et al. Subscription to the surgical council on resident education web portal and qualifying exam performance. J Am Coll Surg 2014;218:566–70.

42. Mayer RE. Applying the science of learning: evidence-based principles for the design of multimedia instruction. Am Psychol 2008;63:760–9.

43. Mayer RE, Mathias A, Wetzell K. Fostering understanding of multi-media message through pre-training: evidence for a two-stage theory of mental model construction. J Exp Psychol Appl 2002;8:147–54.

44. About Med U. Med U Web site. 2013. Available at: http://www.med-u.org/about/our-history/our-story. Accessed June 23, 2015.

45. Phitayakorn R, Nick MW, Alseidi A, et al. WISE-MD usage among millennial medical students. Am J Surg 2015;209:152–7.

46. WebSurg- the e-surgical reference. WebSurg Web site. 2015. Available at: http://www.websurg.com/about_us/. Accessed June 23, 2015.

47. Glass NE, Kulaylat AN, Zheng F, et al. A national survey of educational resources utilized by the Resident and Associate Society of the American College of Surgeons membership. Am J Surg 2015;209:59–64.

48. Barry DS, Marzouk F, Chulak-Oglu K, et al. Anatomy education for the YouTube generation. Anat Sci Educ 2015. http://www.dx.doi.org/10.1002/ase.1550. [Epub ahead of print].

49. Podcast - Definition and more from the Free Merriam-Webster Dictionary. 2012. Available at: Merriam-webster.com. Accessed June 29, 2015.

50. White JS, Sharma N, Boora P. Surgery 101: evaluating the use of podcasting in a general surgery clerkship. Med Teach 2011;33:941–3.

51. Farooq A, White J. No more textbooks? The impact of rapid communications technologies on medical education. Can J Surg 2014;57:E119–20.

52. Kaplan AM, Haenlein M. Users of the world, unite! The challenges and opportunities of social media. Bus Horiz 2010;53:61.

53. Cheston CC, Flickinger TE, Chisolm MS. Social media use in medical education: a systematic review. Acad Med 2013;88:893–901.

54. Aristotle quotes. Brainy Quote Web site. Available at: http://www.brainyquote.com/quotes/quotes/a/aristotle145967.html. Accessed July 1, 2015.

55. Dreyfus HL, Dreyfus SE. Mind over machine: the power of human intuition and expertise in the era of the computer. New York: The Free Press; 1986.

56. De Leo G, Diggs LA, Radici E, et al. Measuring sense of presence and user characteristics to predict effective training in an online simulated virtual environment. Simul Healthc 2014;9:1–6.

57. Olasky J, Sankaranarayanan G, Seymour NE, et al. Identifying opportunities for virtual reality simulation in surgical education: a review of the proceedings from the Innovation, Design and Emerging Alliances in Surgery (IDEAS) Conference: VR Surgery. Surg Innov 2015;22(5):514–21.

58. Halvorsen FH, Elle OJ, Fosse E. Simulators in surgery. Minim Invasive Ther Allied Technol 2005;14:214–23.

59. Pelligrini CA. Surgical education in the United States: navigating the white waters. Ann Surg 2006;244:335–42.

60. Dutta S, Gaba D, Krummel TM. To simulate or not to simulate: what is the question? Ann Surg 2006;243:301–3.
61. Tang LW, D'Ancona G, Bergsland J, et al. Robotically assisted video-enhanced-endoscopic coronary artery bypass graft surgery. Angiology 2001;52:99–102.
62. Hanzly MI, Al-Tartir T, Raza SJ, et al. Simulation-based training in robot-assisted surgery: current evidence of value and potential trends for the future. Curr Urol Rep 2015;16:41.
63. Liu A, Tendick F, Cleary K, et al. A survey of surgical simulation: applications, technology, and education. Presence 2003;12:599–614.
64. Calatayud D, Arora S, Aggarwal R, et al. Warm-up in a virtual reality environment improves performance in the operating room. Ann Surg 2010;251:1181–5.
65. Lee J, Mucksavage P, Kerbl D, et al. Laparoscopic warm-up exercises improve performance of senior-level trainees during laparoscopic renal surgery. J Endourol 2012;26:545.
66. Rassweiler J, Binder J, Frede T. Robotic and telesurgery: will they change our future? Curr Opin Urol 2001;11:309–20.
67. Society of American Gastrointestinal Endoscopic Surgeons. Guidelines for the surgical practices of telemedicine. Surg Endosc 2000;14:975–9.
68. Huie SS. Facilitating telemedicine: reconciling national access with state licensing laws. Hastings Comm Entertain Law J 1995;18:377.
69. Eliasson AH, Poropatich RK. Performance improvement in telemedicine: essential elements. Mil Med 1998;163:530–5.
70. Allen D, Bowersox J, Jones GG. Telesurgery. Telepresence. Telemonitoring. Tele-robotics. Telemed Today 1997;5(3):18–20, 25.
71. Link RE, Schulam PG, Kavoussi LR. Telesurgery. Remote monitoring and assistance during laparoscopy. Urol Clin North Am 2001;28:177–88.
72. Kaplan SJ, Carroll JT, Nematollahi S, et al. Utilization of a non-preserved cadaver to address deficiencies in technical skills during the third year of medical school: a cadaver model for teaching technical skills. World J Surg 2013;37:953–5.
73. Haluck RS, Krummel TM. Computers and virtual reality for surgical education the in the 21st century. Arch Surg 2000;135:786–91.
74. Issenberg SB, McGaghie WE, Hart IR, et al. Simulation technology for health care professional skills training and assessment. JAMA 1999;282:861–6.
75. Rosser JC, Laynch P, Cuddihy L, et al. The impact of video games on training surgeons in the 21st century. Arch Surg 2007;142:181–6.
76. Adams BJ, Margaron F, Kaplan BJ. Comparing video games and laparoscopic simulators in the development of laparoscopic skills in surgical residents. J Surg Educ 2012;69:714–7.
77. Towle Millard HA, Millard RP, Constable PD, et al. Relationships among video gaming proficiency and spatial orientation, laparoscopic and traditional surgical skills of third-year veterinary students. J Am Vet Med Assoc 2014;244:357–62.
78. Lin DT, Park J, Liebert CA, et al. Validity evidence for surgical improvement of clinical knowledge ops: a novel gaming platform to assess surgical decision making. Am J Surg 2015;209:79–85.
79. Quotes about excess. Goodreads Web site. Available at: http://www.goodreads.com/quotes/tag/excess. Accessed June 23, 2015.
80. Kuznekoff JH, Titsworth S. The impact of mobile phone usage on student learning. Commun Educ 2013;62:233–52.
81. Kraushaar JM, Novak DC. Examining the effects of student multitasking with laptops during the lecture. J Info Syst Educ 2010;21:241–51.

82. Ophir E, Nass C, Wagner AD. Cognitive control in media multitaskers. Proc Natl Acad Sci U S A 2009;106(37):15583–7.
83. Taylor J. Technology: myth of multitasking. Psychology Today Web site. 2011. Available at: http://www.psychologytoday.com/blog/the-power-prime/201103/technology-myth-multitasking. Accessed July 1, 2015.
84. Boruff JT, Storie D. Mobile devices in medicine: a survey of how medical students, residents and faculty use smartphones and other mobile devices to find information. J Med Libr Assoc 2014;102:22–30.
85. Ozdalga E, Ozdalga A, Ahuja N. The smartphone in medicine: a review of current and potential use among physicians and students. J Med Internet Res 2012;14: e128.
86. Mobasheri MH, Johnston M, Syed UM, et al. The uses of smartphones and tablet devices in surgery: a systematic review of the literature. Surgery 2015. http://dx.doi.org/10.1016/j.surg.2015.03.029. [Epub ahead of print].
87. Sclafani J, Tirrell TF, Franko OI. Mobile tablet use among academic physicians and trainees. J Med Syst 2013;37:9903.
88. Shah D, Galante JM, Bold RJ, et al. Text messaging among residents and faculty in a university general surgery residency program: prevalence, purpose, and patient care. J Surg Educ 2013;70:827–34.

The Impaired Surgeon

Ranjan Sudan, MD*, Keri Seymour, DO

KEYWORDS

- Impaired • Physician • Alcohol • Drugs

KEY POINTS

- Impaired physicians commonly refers to those who suffer from substance use disorders (SUDs).
- The annual prevalence is approximately 10% to 12%.
- Treatment is available through physician health programs (PHPs).
- Prognosis for recovery and preservation of the ability to practice medicine are excellent for more than 70% of the participants.

BACKGROUND

According to the American Medical Association (AMA), an impaired physician is one whose physical or mental health interferes with their ability to engage safely in professional activities.[1] Such impairment can be the result of a substance use disorder (SUD), mental health issues, or physical health problems. Although by this definition "physician impairment" can be used broadly, it is more commonly used to describe a physician who has a SUD and is the focus of this article.

Previously, substance abuse and substance dependence were 2 separate diagnostic categories. The *Diagnostic and Statistical Manual of Mental Disorders* (Fifth Edition), however, combined them into a single disorder that is measured on a continuum from mild to severe, and each specific substance use is addressed separately (eg, alcohol use disorder). To diagnose SUDs, 11 symptoms are assessed that relate to impaired control, social impairment, risky use, and pharmacologic criteria, such as tolerance and withdrawal. In general, a mild SUD is suggested by the presence of 2 to 3 symptoms, moderate by 4 to 5 symptoms, and severe by 6 or more symptoms. These include taking the substance in larger amounts and for longer period than intended; wanting to cut down or stop using the substance but not being able to; spending a lot of time getting or recovering from use of the substance; craving and urges to use the substance; not keeping up with work or school because of substance

Disclosure Statement: The authors have nothing to disclose.
Department of Surgery, Duke University Medical Center, Box 2834, Durham, NC 27710, USA
* Corresponding author.
E-mail address: Ranjan.sudan@duke.edu

use; continuing to use the substance even when it is causing problems in relation-ships; giving up important social, occupational, or recreational activities because of substance use; using substances repeatedly even when it puts a person in danger; continuing substance use despite the knowledge that physical or psychological prob-lems have been caused or made worse by the substance; and needing more sub-stance to get the effect (tolerance) or the development of withdrawal symptoms.

Prevalence

In the United States, the 12-month prevalence of alcohol use disorder in the general population is estimated to be 8.5% among adults age 18 years and older with greater rates among adult men (12.4%) than among adult women (4.9%).[2] Many studies es-timate that the rate of alcohol use disorder in physicians parallels that of the general community and the factors that predispose individuals to SUDs are similar among physicians and the general population. Certain factors are unique to physicians such as easier access, knowledge of the medications, and the ability to prescribe, which predispose to higher use of opioids, benzodiazepines, fentanyl, and propofol, particularly in certain specialties, such as anesthesia and psychiatry.[3–10]

Despite similar prevalences of SUDs among physicians and the general population, physicians are held to a higher standard because of the trust that society has placed in them to make critical life-and-death decisions for patients and their conduct has the potential to impact the quality and safety of health care delivered. Therefore, SUDs have far-reaching consequences not only for physicians and their own families but also on the work environment and the patients they treat.

Impairment Is Treatable

In recognition of the impact that impairment has on physicians and on their commu-nity, a landmark article was published in the Journal of the American Medical Associ-ation in 1973 by the AMA Council on Mental Health, "The Sick Physician: Impairment by Psychiatric Disorders, Including Alcoholism and Drug Dependence."[11] The work of this council led the AMA to acknowledge physician impairment in 1974, recognizing alcoholism and other SUDs as illnesses and suggesting alternate ways of managing them other than through disciplinary actions, and eventually led to the development of physician health programs (PHP) in all states. Prior to that, the Federation of State Medical Boards identified drug addiction and alcoholism among doctors primarily as disciplinary problems and very few states had programs in place to treat impaired phy-sicians. PHPs are now available in every state and are administered either by the state medical boards or the medical societies. The Federation of State Physician Health Programs is a forum for exchange of information among these various programs that seeks to standardize their goals and objectives. It is also engaged in advocacy for impaired physicians while at the same time safeguarding the public.

A physician may either self-refer or be referred to a PHP by a colleague or a medical staff office. Entering a contractual agreement with a PHP helps impaired physicians get appropriate treatment confidentially, allowing them to keep their license and subse-quently practice, after completing treatment. Thus, formal disciplinary action is avoided while they obtain treatment. Typically, PHPs do not themselves provide treatment but they do provide early detection, assessment, evaluation, and referral to selected treat-ment facilities. Many of these facilities provide residential treatment for 60 to 90 days followed by a 12-step–oriented outpatient treatment program that includes frequent random drug and alcohol testing along with workplace monitors. The reports of these evaluations are then provided to appropriate credentialing authorities, such as hospi-tals, malpractice companies, and health insurance companies for 5 or more years.

This reporting system allows the participant to practice while simultaneously protecting patients and coworkers. Operating funds for a PHP come from state licensing boards, participant fees, state medical associations, hospital contributions, and malpractice companies. A mean of 34 physicians enter a PHP each year. On entering, the participant must sign a contract that provides the specifics of treatment and monitoring and the consequences of not adhering to this contract. PHPs do not have the authority to discipline physicians but they can make recommendations to state licensure boards that could result in severe disciplinary repercussions. Preservation of license and the ability to practice are, therefore, strong motivators for physicians to stay engaged in the program.[12,13] Several studies have shown that more than 70% of the physicians going through a PHP were able to stay in practice 5 years later.

IDENTIFYING AN IMPAIRED PHYSICIAN

The AMA has now made it an ethical obligation to report impaired colleagues in accordance with the legal requirements of each state to ensure that impaired physicians cease practice and receive appropriate assistance from a PHP. Identifying an impaired colleague has its challenges, because physicians are good at hiding their substance use and often the problem has to be severe before it is discovered. Some authors have recommended mandatory testing for drugs and alcohol after a sentinel event such as after an accident in the airline or transportation industry.[14] More often, deteriorating social and interpersonal behaviors are first noticed by friends and family. In the work environment, inaccessibility to patients and staff, unexplained absenteeism, frequent conflicts with coworkers, and frequent moves to different locations for jobs may be warning signs.[15] Certainly, the smell of alcohol on a person's breath or impaired motor coordination at work cannot be ignored. Comorbid mental disorders are also common in physicians with SUDs and are associated with a higher relapse rate. Major depression, bipolar disorder, social phobia, generalized anxiety disorder, and antisocial personality disorder were among the more common diagnoses identified in impaired physicians and may also predispose towards suicide.[16,17]

Although such symptoms are noticed by peers, they are reluctant to report an impaired colleague or a friend to the appropriate authorities. The desire to avoid confrontation or fear of damaging a physician's career, especially when the signs and symptoms are subtle, is among the stated reasons for this reluctance.[18] It is an ethical obligation, however, and in most states a legal requirement, that physicians report impaired colleagues to the state medical boards or PHPs. The PHPs then undertake suitable in-depth evaluation and make further recommendations.

INTERVENING WITH AN IMPAIRED PHYSICIAN

Colleagues should not diagnose or treat an individual with an SUD. Instead, they should record details of the behavior and performance suggestive of an SUD. Presenting these facts becomes important when performing an 'intervention' with an impaired physician. An *intervention* is the formal process of presenting these facts and is led by an experienced individual. Friends, families, and coworkers can also be involved in the intervention. It is imperative that all the participants be unanimous in their belief that the physician is impaired and needs help. The urgency with which this intervention is delivered needs to be individualized based on the severity of the symptoms and the need to provide a safe environment for coworkers and patients. The implementation of the action plan must be immediate. When faced with such an intervention, many impaired physicians agree to an evaluation through a PHP or risk being reported to the state board and facing disciplinary action, such as losing their license to practice medicine. Should an impaired physician deny the problem or even become belligerent, then the individuals who are engaged in the intervention should have contingency plans for addressing these scenarios. It is reassuring that the most common sources of referrals to PHPs are self-referrals (26%). Other referring sources include state licensing boards (20%), hospital medical staff (14%), and miscellaneous sources, such as law enforcement, medical schools, family members, and lawyers (17%). Only a minority of the participants entered a PHP after a formal stipulation from a regulatory authority.[12,13]

OUTCOMES

Overall the outcomes of physicians undergoing treatment and extended monitoring for substance use are excellent and better than in the general population, which most likely represents their motivation to maintain their license and practice medicine with its associated financial and social rewards. Relapses are considered breaches of contract and include reusing the prohibited substance and noncompliance with program requirements, such as missing meetings or drug testing or other behavioral concerns. Noncompliance is dealt with aggressively and, depending on severity, penalties may vary from increased monitoring to discontinuation of work and reevaluation or additional treatment.

A study of 63 impaired physicians in Oregon who were followed-up for 8 years in a rehabilitation program for repetitive drug abuse showed that 75% were rated as stable and improved. Those subjects who were monitored with random urine screens for drug use were more successful (96%) compared with those who were treated but not monitored with random screening (64%), suggesting that random urine monitoring during a 2-year to 4-year period is positively correlated with treatment outcome.[19]

In another study of 904 physicians from 16 PHPs, 631 participants (78.7%) were licensed and working, 87 (10.8%) had their licenses revoked, 28 (3.5%) had retired, 30 (3.7%) had died, and 26 (3.2%) had unknown status, suggesting overall positive outcomes.[6] A subgroup of this larger cohort was surgeons and their results were compared with nonsurgeons. Overall, surgeons had positive outcomes that were similar to nonsurgeons.[20]

This remarkable rate of success for physicians treated through PHPs is considerably higher than that of the general population, which has relapse rates of 40% to 60%. The reasons for the success of PHPs were investigated in a survey of 42 such programs. Results showed that all of the PHPs had similar goals. Evaluation and treatment strategies included working with professional societies, medical centers, professional colleagues, friends, and families to evaluate and treat impaired physicians. An essential part of the treatment was a signed contract and referral to carefully selected residential facilities where the treatment was individualized and was followed by a sustained period of monitoring that included frequent random drug testing and engagement of the participant's support system. Protection from adverse licensing and legal actions while a physician was participating in a PHP was also a powerful motivator. Most other substance abuse programs do not offer the intensity, individualization, and prolonged monitoring offered by PHPs and are, therefore, less likely to be successful.[21,22]

SUMMARY

Impaired physicians harm themselves, their families, patients, coworkers, and institutions. It is an ethical and legal obligation to report such individuals and facilitate their opportunities for recovery. Such help is available through PHPs, and the prognosis for participants in such programs to recover and practice medicine is excellent.

REFERENCES

1. Available at: http://www.ama-assn.org/ama/pub/physician-resources/medical-ethics/code-medical-ethics/opinion90305. Accessed September 1, 2015.
2. Diagnostic and statistical manual of mental disorders-5. Washington, DC: American Psychiatric Association; 2013.
3. McAuliffe WE, Rohman M, Breer P, et al. Alcohol use and abuse in random samples of physicians and medical students. Am J Public Health 1991;81(2):177–82.
4. Niven RG, Hurt RD, Morse RM, et al. Alcoholism in physicians. Mayo Clin Proc 1984;59(1):12–6.
5. McGovern MP, Angres DH, Leon S. Characteristics of physicians presenting for assessment at a behavioral health center. J Addict Dis 2000;19(2):59–73.
6. McLellan AT, Skipper GS, Campbell M, et al. Five year outcomes in a cohort study of physicians treated for substance use disorders in the United States. BMJ 2008; 337:a2038.
7. Hughes PH, Storr CL, Brandenburg NA, et al. Physician substance use by medical specialty. J Addict Dis 1999;18(2):23–37.
8. Brewster JM. Prevalence of alcohol and other drug problems among physicians. JAMA 1986;255(14):1913–20.
9. Hughes PH, Brandenburg N, Baldwin DC Jr, et al. Prevalence of substance use among US physicians. JAMA 1992;267(17):2333–9.
10. McAuliffe WE, Rohman M, Santangelo S, et al. Psychoactive drug use among practicing physicians and medical students. N Engl J Med 1986;315(13):805–10.
11. The sick physician. Impairment by psychiatric disorders, including alcoholism and drug dependence. JAMA 1973;223(6):684–7.
12. DuPont RL, McLellan AT, Carr G, et al. How are addicted physicians treated? A national survey of Physician Health Programs. J Subst Abuse Treat 2009;37(1):1–7.
13. DuPont RL, McLellan AT, White WL, et al. Setting the standard for recovery: physicians' health programs. J Subst Abuse Treat 2009;36(2):159–71.
14. Pham JC, Pronovost PJ, Skipper GE. Identification of physician impairment. JAMA 2013;309(20):2101–2.
15. Breiner SJ. The impaired physician. J Med Educ 1979;54(8):673.
16. Cottler LB, Ajinkya S, Merlo LJ, et al. Lifetime psychiatric and substance use disorders among impaired physicians in a physicians health program: comparison to a general treatment population: psychopathology of impaired physicians. J Addict Med 2013;7(2):108–12.
17. Wijesinghe CP, Dunne F. Substance use and other psychiatric disorders in impaired practitioners. Psychiatr Q 2001;72(2):181–9.
18. Farber NJ, Gilibert SG, Aboff BM, et al. Physicians' willingness to report impaired colleagues. Soc Sci Med 2005;61(8):1772–5.
19. Shore JH. The Oregon experience with impaired physicians on probation. An eight-year follow-up. JAMA 1987;257(21):2931–4.
20. Buhl A, Oreskovich MR, Meredith CW, et al. Prognosis for the recovery of surgeons from chemical dependency: a 5-year outcome study. Arch Surg 2011; 146(11):1286–91.
21. Finney JW, Ouimette PC, Humphreys K, et al. A comparative, process-effectiveness evaluation of VA substance abuse treatment. Recent Dev Alcohol 2001;15:373–91.
22. Weisner C, Mertens J, Parthasarathy S, et al. The outcome and cost of alcohol and drug treatment in an HMO: day hospital versus traditional outpatient regimens. Health Serv Res 2000;35(4):791–812.

Workforce Needs and Demands in Surgery

Chandrakanth Are, MD, MBA, FRCS

KEYWORDS

- Surgical training • Graduate medical education • General surgery
- Surgical workforce

KEY POINTS

- The rapidly evolving health care environment will place enormous pressure on the surgical training systems of today and thereby influence the surgical workforce of tomorrow.
- Despite the controversy about the workforce adequacy, it is highly probable that we will face a shortage of general surgeons or surgeons that perform general surgical procedures in the future.
- It is unlikely that the surgical workforce of the future can be augmented without significantly increasing the number of residency positions which seems improbable in the current environment.
- The surgical community needs to demonstrate strong leadership to develop innovative models of graduate medical education that will ensure an adequate surgical workforce for the future.

INTRODUCTION

Around the turn of 19th century, William Stewart Halsted, (**Fig. 1**) the first surgeon-in-chief at The Johns Hopkins Hospital, was laying the foundation of what would become one of the most durable models of postgraduate training for physicians in the history of medical education. The existing systems of that time consisted of apprentice models of varying types with no consistency in length, structure, supervision, or assessment of competency prior to entering practice. Halsted's dissatisfaction with the existing systems, combined with the knowledge he acquired during his European travels, sowed the seeds for the Halstedian model. This model consisted of a structured training model over a finite period of time with supervision and progressive assumption of increasing responsibility until acquisition of competence prior to entering practice.

The attractiveness of this model and proven efficacy led to its approval by the American Medical Association House of Delegates in 1928 as the preferred model

Disclosures: None.
Department of Surgery, 986345, University of Nebraska Medical Center, Omaha, NE 68198, USA
E-mail address: care@unmc.edu

Surg Clin N Am 96 (2016) 95–113
http://dx.doi.org/10.1016/j.suc.2015.09.007
0039-6109/16/$ – see front matter © 2016 Elsevier Inc. All rights reserved.

surgical.theclinics.com

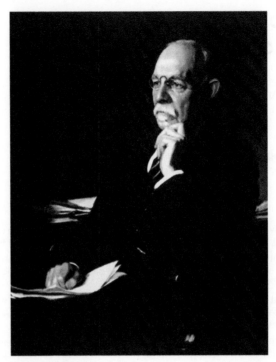

Fig. 1. Dr William Stewart Halsted.

for approving hospital-based residencies in specialties.[1] The resilience of this model is demonstrated by the fact that not only did it become the platform for surgical training, but for training in all specialties, and with some minor modifications, it is the predominant model for training postgraduate physicians worldwide.

The past 2 decades have brought forth more changes to the field of surgery than the entire previous century. This includes the introduction of minimally invasive techniques, adoption of duty hour rules and regulations, new regulations driven by elected officials and the public, demands for delivering value for the investments in graduate medical education, and changing sociocultural fabric with increasing population of greater linguistic diversity. Although the Halstedian model still holds value, surgical training models of the future need to demonstrate preternatural flexibility to adapt to the unending cycle of change and still produce surgeons of competence. This is extremely important, since good surgical training pathways of today contribute to pipelines that generate the surgical workforce of tomorrow.

An adequate surgical workforce is the core requirement to provide adequate surgical services to any nation. An ideal surgical workforce should consist of an adequate number of competent surgeons trained across all specialties that is distributed on a needs basis across the entire nation. Several concerns have been raised in recent times about the competence of trainees, adequacy of graduates, and the uneven distribution of surgical workforce across the nation. Concerns such as these about the workforce lead to question the validity of current surgical training paradigms and whether they are structured to meet the workforce needs of the future. Unless one addresses the issues burdening the surgical training systems of today, the problems associated with the surgical workforce of tomorrow will go unsolved.

The aims of this article are to

1. Develop an understanding of the definitions and dynamics of surgical workforce and provide an overview of the current trends/issues in surgical workforce
2. Present the current model of training from medical school to practice with some suggested changes to the training system of today to address issues with the surgical workforce of tomorrow; for the purposes of this article, the focus will be placed on training during general surgery residency and workforce of general surgeons.

DEFINITIONS AND DYNAMICS OF SURGICAL WORKFORCE AND OVERVIEW OF CURRENT TRENDS AND ISSUES
Current Workforce Data

Workforce is defined as "the people engaged in or available for work, either in a country or area or in a particular company or industry."[2] The Bureau of Labor Statistics documented that the number of jobs for physicians and surgeons in the year 2012 equaled 691,400.[3] This figure is approximately similar to the data published by the American College of Surgeons Health Policy Research Institute (ACS HPRI), which noted the total number of physicians for the year 2009 to be 694,843.[4] Further analysis by ACS HPRI reveals data on the surgical workforce as outlined in **Table 1**. There are 28,926 general surgeons, accounting for approximately 4.1% of the physician workforce in the nation.

Change in Workforce Numbers

The change in workforce numbers between the years 2005 and 2009 is outlined in **Table 2**[4] and reveals alarming trends for the general surgeon workforce. Although general surgery subspecialties witnessed a growth of nearly 21%, the growth in general surgery alone stood at 0.2%.[4] General surgery subspecialties consisted of abdominal surgery, surgical critical care, hand surgery, oral and maxillofacial surgery, pediatric surgery, surgical oncology, trauma surgery, transplant surgery, vascular surgery, cardiovascular surgery, and pediatric surgical subspecialties.

Distribution of the Surgical Workforce in the United States

The American College of Surgeons Health Policy Institute provides data on distribution of the surgical workforce based on the number of counties.[5] The data are categorized as 2 groups: all surgeons and general surgeons only, and is provided as the number of

Table 1
Physician/Surgeon workforce in the United States for 2009

Specialty		Total Active Physicians
All specialties		694,843
All surgical specialties		135,854
General surgery	Composite[a]	28,926
	General surgery alone	22,486
	General surgery subspecialties	6440

[a] Composite = General surgery alone + general surgery subspecialties.

Data from The surgical workforce in the United States: profile and recent trends. American College of Surgeons Health Policy Research Institute. Available at: http://www.acshpri.org/documents/ACSHPRI_Surgical_Workforce_in_US_apr2010.pdf. Accessed June 14, 2015.

Table 2
Percentage change in the surgical workforce for 2009 when compared with 2005

	Specialty	Total Active Physicians (% Change)
All specialties		+ 7.8%
All surgical specialties		+ 2.6%
General surgery	Composite[a]	+ 4.2%
	General surgery alone	+ 0.2%
	General surgery subspecialties	+ 20.9%

[a] Composite = General surgery alone + general surgery subspecialties.
Data from The surgical workforce in the United States: profile and recent trends. American College of Surgeons Health Policy Research Institute. Available at: http://www.acshpri.org/documents/ACSHPRI_Surgical_Workforce_in_US_apr2010.pdf. Accessed June 14, 2015.

surgeons per 100,000 population in each county within the United States. The data include nonfederal, nonresident, clinically active physicians less than 80 years of age reporting their primary specialty as "surgery" or "general surgery."These data, revised on Oct. 12, 2012, cover the period from 2006 to 2011 and are summarized in **Table 3**. Although the pattern of uneven distribution is evident nationwide for all surgical specialties, this trend is much worse for the distribution of general surgeons. The number of counties with at least 40 general surgeons decreased by almost 33%. Although 128 counties gained a general surgeon in 2011 when compared with 2006, a greater number of counties (206) completely lost all general surgeons.

Table 3
Distribution of surgical workforce in the United States based on the number of counties

Number of Surgeons in 2006 and 2011			
		All Surgeons/1000,000 Population	General Surgeons Only/100,000 Population
Number of counties with ≥40 surgeons	2006	679	12
	2011	668	8
Number of counties with 0.1–4.6 surgeons	2006	84	324
	2011	100	386
Number of counties with no surgeons	2006	841	1066
	2011	898	1144

% Change in Number of Surgeons/100,000 Population Between 2006 and 2011		
	All Surgeons	General Surgeons Only
Number of counties that gained 100% or more surgeons	90	88
Number of counties with no change	1	0
Number of counties with decline in number of surgeons	1051	1139
No surgeons in 2006 but at least 1 surgeon in 2011	136	128
Number of counties that lost all surgeons	193	206

Data from Distribution of surgical workforce in the United States, American College of Surgeons Health Policy Institute. Available at: http://www.acshpri.org/documents/SurgeonMaps2006-2011_Oct2012.pdf. Accessed June 21, 2015.

Number of Some of the Common General Surgical Procedures Performed in the United States

The US Centers for Disease Control and Prevention documented that 51.4 million procedures were performed in the United States in 2010 based on the National Hospital Discharge Survey.[6] Because this includes a large number of nongeneral surgical procedures such as joint replacements, cesarean section, and cardiac catheterization, further attempts were made to determine the number of general surgical procedures performed annually in the United States. A review of the National Hospital Discharge Survey[7] documented the data for some common general surgical procedures from short-stay hospitals as outlined in **Table 4**. These data are far from accurate, as they do not include several other common procedures such as hernia repair, and are unlikely to capture data from all in-patient or day-procedure settings. Nonetheless these data provide an approximate measure of the number of some of the common general surgical procedures performed in the United States.

Population Growth in the United States

The number of general surgeons needed to address the surgical needs of the nation is directly proportional to the population. The population growth trends for the United States for the next 45 years are outlined in **Table 5**.[8] Although the percentage increase shows a decreasing trend, it is noted that the population of United States will increase by an additional 95 million by the year 2060. This increase in the population will most certainly increase the number of general surgical procedures, and thereby increase the need for general surgeons. A 10-year update study by Valentine and colleagues[9] on general surgery workloads documented an increase in the number of cases performed by general surgeons annually from 398 cases (reporting period from 1995 to 1997) to 533 (reporting period from 2007 to 2009). Although not analyzed in the study, the population of the United States increased in the corresponding time period from 266,490,000 in 1997[10] to 296,824,000 in 2007,[11] mirroring the increased number of surgical procedures documented by Valentine and colleagues.

Pipeline for Training General Surgeons

The trends in the number of positions offered for general surgery residency in the matching program for the last 25 years are shown in **Fig. 2**.[12] We noticed a decrease in the number of positions, saddling around the turn of the millennium, with a slight increase in the numbers of positions in most the recent 5-year period. Nonetheless,

Table 4
Number of routine general surgical procedures performed in the United States in 2010

Type of Procedure	# of Procedures	Standard Error
Partial excision of large intestine	247,000	30
Appendectomy, excluding incidental	305,000	46
Cholecystectomy	429,000	47
Lysis of peritoneal adhesions	356,000	43
Total	1,337,000	—

Data from Center for Disease Control and Prevention. National Hospital Discharge Surgery: 2010 table, procedures by selected patient characteristics—number by procedure category and age. Available at: http://www.cdc.gov/nchs/data/nhds/4procedures/2010pro4_numberprocedureage.pdf. Accessed June 14, 2015.

Table 5
Population projections for the United States

Year	Population (in Thousands)	Approximate % Increase
2015	321,369	–
2025	347,335	8%
2035	370,338	6.6%
2045	389,394	5.1%
2055	407,412	4.6%
2060	416,795	2.2%

Data from United States Census Bureau, Population Projections. 2014 national population projections: summary tables. Available at: http://www.census.gov/population/projections/data/national/2014/summarytables.html. Accessed June 14, 2015.

these changes remain modest and are extremely unlikely to alter the number of graduates and therefore the workforce in any significant fashion.

The interpretation of the previously described data leads to several objective findings:

1. The population of United States is expected to rise significantly.
2. The number of general surgical procedures performed will likely rise.
3. The number of procedures performed by general surgeons is already on the rise.
4. The surgical workforce data demonstrate that the number of general surgeons has remained static, whereas there has been a 20% increase in the number of surgeons in general surgery subspecialties.
5. There is an uneven distribution of the surgical workforce in the United States, with the trends being even more worrisome for general surgeons.
6. The number of training positions in general surgery has not changed significantly over the past 25 years, and therefore the current training model is unlikely to increase the workforce numbers in the near future.

From the previously described data and findings, it appears that there will be a shortage of general surgeons in the future. Although this may seem straightforward from the data provided here, the debate on the topic of physician and general surgeon shortage is conflicting. Public and policy debate on the topic is highly contradictory, which makes it nearly impossible to reach clear and cogent conclusions. Another cause for confusion is the cross-referencing of data on supply and demand between the different specialties, which can lead to misinterpretation of the published findings.

To reach some consensus for this article, reports on physician supply and demand published by one agency, the Bureau of Health Professions, Health Resources and Services Administration (BPHR, HRSA) with be used. The article will refer to sequential reports published by HRSA on physician supply and demand over the last decade (**Table 6**). Although these reports are published by the same agency, review of the variable findings in the sequential reports illustrates the difficulty in accurately projecting the supply demand curves for the future.

The HRSA published a report on "Physician Supply and Demand: Projections to 2020" in October 2006, which stated that the overall physician supply per capita will remain relatively stable for the next 15 years.[13] By using the Physician Supply Model (PSM) and Physician Requirement Model (PRM) the report summarized that the overall supply of physicians should be sufficient to meet the expected demand through the next 10 years until 2016. An updated report published in December 2008[14] noted

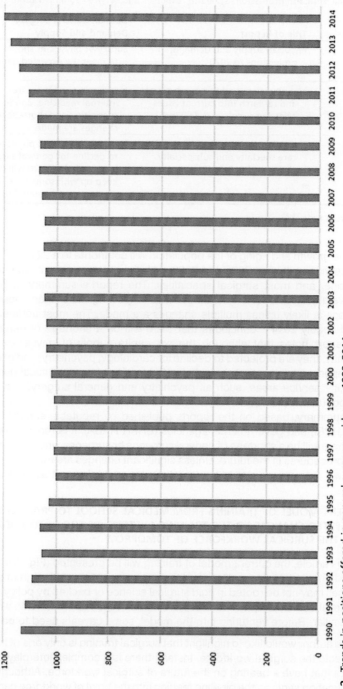

Fig. 2. Trends in positions offered in general surgery residency: 1990–2014.

Table 6
Data on projections of general surgery supply and demand based on reports published by bureau of health professionals, health resources and services administration: 2006 to 2014

Year Published	Title of Report	Data on General Surgery Demand and Supply
2006	Physician supply and demand: projections to 2020[13]	Supply of physicians should be sufficient to meet the expected demand through 2016
2008	The physician workforce: projections and research into current issues affecting supply and demand[14]	Increase in need is greatest in cardiology, internal medicine, and surgical specialties; and shortage is likely unless changes are made
2014	Projecting the supply of nonprimary care specialty and subspecialty clinicians: 2010–2015[15]	Per capita supply of physicians projected to decline for general surgery, and supply of physicians will not be able to keep up with some specialties such as psychiatry and general surgery

Data from Refs.[13–15]

that the growth and aging of the population will contribute to a 22% increase in physician services between 2005 and 2020, with the greatest need in cardiology, internal medicine, and most surgical specialties. The report's summary documented that the overall demand for physician services is growing faster than supply, implying a shortage is likely unless multiple changes are made. The most updated report published in July 2014[15] concludes that there will be a shortage of general surgeons. The report notes that although the per capita supply of physicians will vary by specialty, they are projected to decline for cardiology, psychiatry, and general surgery. The report concludes that the supply of physicians in some critical nonprimary care specialty service areas, such as psychiatry and general surgery, may not keep up with population growth.

In summary, based on the reports published by reputable surgical organizations (ACS HPRI) and governmental agencies (BHPR HRSA), it is reasonable to conclude that there will be a shortage of general surgeons or surgeons who perform general surgical procedures in the future. Unless significant changes are made now, these shortages will only worsen due to the long time period it takes to train general surgeons.

CURRENT MODEL OF TRAINING FROM MEDICAL SCHOOL TO PRACTICE WITH SOME SUGGESTED CHANGES TO THE TRAINING SYSTEMS OF TODAY TO ADDRESS ISSUES WITH THE SURGICAL WORKFORCE OF TOMORROW

For this article, the current model of training will be presented (**Fig. 3**) with some suggested changes to some stages of this training paradigm. Although many suggested changes may not be rooted in rigid surgical science or backed by policy metrics, most readers should be acquainted with the common sense approach with which surgeons are familiar. Before venturing into the model, some caveats need to be highlighted:

1. The author would like to highlight that surgical training is only one of the factors that affects the surgical workforce. Instead there is a complex interplay of several factors that have a bearing on the future of surgical workforce. Although training and education serve as the pipeline feeding into the bowl of workforce capacity, several post-training factors play a more significant role.

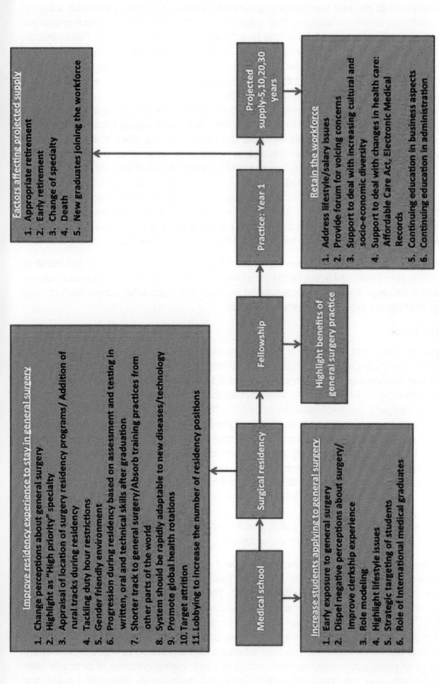

Fig. 3. Current model from medical school to practice with some suggested changes.

Factors affecting projected supply
1. Appropriate retirement
2. Early retirement
3. Change of specialty
4. Death
5. New graduates joining the workforce

Improve residency experience to stay in general surgery
1. Change perceptions about general surgery
2. Highlight as "High priority" specialty
3. Appraisal of location of surgery residency programs/ Addition of rural tracks during residency
4. Tackling duty hour restrictions
5. Gender friendly environment
6. Progression during residency based on assessment and testing in written, oral and technical skills after graduation
7. Shorter track to general surgery/Absorb training practices from other parts of the world
8. System should be rapidly adaptable to new diseases/technology
9. Promote global health rotations
10. Target attrition
11. Lobbying to increase the number of residency positions

Increase students applying to general surgery
1. Early exposure to general surgery
2. Dispel negative perceptions about surgery/ Improve clerkship experience
3. Role modeling
4. Highlight lifestyle issues
5. Strategic targeting of students
6. Role of International medical graduates

Retain the workforce
1. Address lifestyle/salary issues
2. Provide forum for voicing concerns
3. Support to deal with increasing cultural and socio-economic diversity
4. Support to deal with changes in health care: Affordable Care Act, Electronic Medical Records
5. Continuing education in business aspects
6. Continuing education in administration

Medical school → Surgical residency → Fellowship → Practice: Year 1 → Projected supply-5,10,20,30 years

Highlight benefits of general surgery practice

2. The scope of practice for a general surgeon is in constant evolution and will continue to do so in the future. Several diseases/procedures that were once in the domain of general surgeon's practice are no longer, such as vascular surgery. In contrast, some procedures that were once in the domain of fellowship-trained surgeons are returning into the fold of a general surgeon's practice. For example, some laparoscopic procedures such as Nissen fundoplication, which were once performed by fellowship-trained surgeons, are now performed by general surgeons in practice with or without additional training. As technology is disseminated more freely, more complex laparoscopic procedures will be performed by surgeons who categorize themselves as general surgeons. The scope of practice for a general surgeon is a highly malleable domain and will continue to cause cross-specialty issues. And this nebulous area of separation between the specialties will always make it difficult to determine the actual number of general surgeons and more importantly who is performing the common general surgical procedures.
3. This model with the suggested changes should by no means be considered as a comprehensive mosaic of solutions to address all issues associated with surgical training or surgical workforce. Instead it should be considered as an initial thought platform that can provide the catapult to initiate debate about how one can shape the future of general surgery training and its resultant workforce.

Review of the model reveals several stages that can have a bearing on the surgical workforce. Emphasis will appropriately be placed on the stages of medical school and residency training. The factors associated with other stages after completion of residency training are briefly mentioned in **Fig. 3**.

Medical School

The primary theme of this stage is to increase the number of US seniors who apply to general surgery residency. The number of US seniors applying to general surgery residency has declined considerably over the last 3 to 4 decades. Review of the data from National Residency Matching Program reveals that the number of US seniors applying to general surgery has decreased by 56% from 12.8% in 1978[16] to 5.6% in 2014.[17] It is beyond the scope of this article to review all the factors contributing to this trend. But suffice it to say that several major changes have taken place in the interim 4 decades such as the emergence of newly independent specialties such as emergency medicine, emphasis on surgical specialties, and coalescence or divergence of domains of practice between specialties. While all of this is true, it still does not conceal the distressing fact that fewer and fewer US seniors are applying to general surgery residency.

Several strategies have been put in place over the last few years to entice more US seniors to apply to general surgery residency.

Early exposure of medical students to the field of general surgery

It is known that for most medical students, their first exposure to a general surgeon may be in their third year of medical school. The first 2 years of medical school are a lost window of opportunity for surgeons to interact with medical students. Several authors[18–21] have published their data on curricula that provide the opportunity to interact with first- and second-year medical students. Are and colleagues[18,19] initiated a new curriculum for first-year medical students that consisted of instruction in management of pancreatic malignancies combined with demonstration of clinically relevant anatomy and pancreaticoduodenectomy by using lightly embalmed cadavers. They noted that nearly 57% of students documented an increase in the likelihood of pursuing a surgical career after watching the surgical demonstration. Patel and colleagues[20] initiated a skills-based curriculum (Surgery Saturday curriculum), targeting the first- and second-year medical students. The number of students planning to apply to surgical residency increased from 42% to 88% prior to and after participation in the Surgery Saturday curriculum. It is easy to be critical of these studies, since they do not follow the linear progression of the students until their match date to see if the increased interest translated to an actual increase in match rate. Haggerty and colleagues[21] addressed this issue by following the student's career path from 2003 to 2012 after instituting an 8-week structured summer research program for second-year medical students. In addition to research productivity, this curriculum led to 52.2% of the students matching into general surgery, which is much higher than their own institutional rate as well as the national match rates.

Dispel negative perceptions about general surgery/improve clerkship experience
Negative perceptions about the field of surgery and surgeons are developed by medical students for various reasons due to the influence from diverse quarters such as the media, preceptors, and classmates.[22] The negative perceptions that preclinical medical students harbor can only be worsened by the experiences during surgical clerkships. Stone and colleagues[23] conducted a survey to identify potential issues that students face during surgical clerkship. The results of their survey document that students perceive intimidation and mistreatment during their surgical clerkships. This included mocking during the operative cases, ridiculing in the presence of others, teaching by humiliation, and physical abuse. These experiences serve as pivotal points that conclusively steer medical students away from ever considering a surgical career. Every attempt should be made to dispel negative perceptions by instituting systematic changes that not only address curricular issues but also ameliorate the prevailing unfavorable culture and attitudes toward medical students.

Role models
Role models play a key role in shaping the career paths of students. Although surgical faculty and residents may underestimate their own influence, applicants and medial students tend to rely on role models for shaping their career paths. Quillin and colleagues[24] conducted a survey of third-year medical students and concluded that surgeons tend to underestimate their influence on medical students entering surgery. Similarly, in a multinational study of 8 countries with 841 respondents, final-year medical students (whether choosing surgery or not as a career) noted that presence of good role models is a strong factor to increase the interest in applying for general surgery residency.[25] The role of a surgeon teacher stretches far beyond the confines of an operating room or class room, and surgeons should be cognizant of the influence they hold on medical students.

Highlight lifestyle issues
For an average medical student in his or her twenties, it can be a daunting task to make a career choice that will affect one's professional life for the next 3 to 4 decades. It is quite common for medical students to see the tree but miss the forest by confusing the lifestyle during residency with lifestyle in practice. The onus is on the surgical community to highlight to potential students interested in surgery that lifestyle during residency does not uniformly translate to the lifestyle in practice. In addition, one should emphasize that residency stretches across a finite period of time (usually 5 years or more if taking time off for research), whereas practice as a surgeon is infinite until retirement. Students need to be appraised not to make decisions against a surgical career based on the lifestyle during the limited period of residency but to make decisions based on the multiple rewards of a surgical career after training. It should

also be pointed out to the students that although surgical careers can be stressful due to the nature of the work involved, the rewards are commensurate with the stress involved.

Small-group discussions directed by surgeons to discuss lifestyle after training can be helpful. Some of the earlier studies noted a higher divorce rate among surgeons when compared to other specialties.[26] The more recent studies have noted that physicians in general lead stable lives. Ly and colleagues[27] performed a retrospective analysis of the divorce rates in various professions by using the US census data from 2008 to 2013 and noted that physicians had a lower divorce rate when compared with other professions (**Table 7**). Female physicians had a higher divorce rate than their male counterparts. Although this study did not analyze divorce rates based on specialty, the overall probability of ever being divorced is lower for physicians when compared with other professions. Similarly, Harms and colleagues[28] conducted a 25-year single-institution analysis of the fate of general surgeons and noted a divorce rate of 21.4%, which is similar to the rate from Ly and colleagues[27] for physicians and lower than for other professions. The onus is on the surgical community to educate medical students that surgeons in practice can lead meaningful and happy lives.

Strategic targeting of residents

With regards to pursuing a surgical career, medical students can be categorized into 3 groups. There is a small group of students who are firmly determined that they will pursue a surgical career, and nothing will dissuade them from following on their career aspirations. Many more students are equally firm that they will not pursue surgery regardless of what is offered or presented to them. In between these 2 groups is a group that is undecided and can be influenced to pursue a surgical career. While ensuring that all students receive sufficient education, it might behoove the surgical community to spend some extra effort on the undecided group by providing positive experiences during surgical clerkship to steer them toward a surgical career.

International medical graduates

The drop in interest amongst US seniors[16,17] toward general surgery has led to general surgery residency positions that are increasingly filled by international medical graduates (IMGs) and graduates from other diverse pathways. The role of IMGs in surgery in the United States continues to evolve with the supply–demand cycles. IMGs serve a role on several fronts to augment the surgical workforce in the United States. This includes filling the preliminary positions and accepting jobs in underserved areas.

Table 7	
Divorce rate in various professions: probability of ever being divorced	
Profession	**Divorce Rate in % (95% Confidence Interval)**
Physicians	24.3 (23.8–24.8)
Dentists	25.2 (24.1–26.3)
Pharmacists	22.9 (22.0–23.8)
Nurses	33.0 (32.6–33.3)
Health care executives	30.9 (30.1–31.8)
Lawyers	26.9 (26.4–27.4)
Nonhealth care professionals	35 (34.9–35.1)

Non-US senior applicants into general surgery residency come from diverse sociocultural backgrounds, which can have a bearing on the surgical workforce of the future. A proactive approach needs to be developed on how to integrate the IMGs to the benefit of the surgical workforce in the United States as well as the applicants who arrive on these shores for various reasons.

The surgical community has done an enormous amount of work to keep the pipelines patent for feeding bright medical students into surgical residencies. Despite all these efforts, there have not been any significant increases in the rate of US seniors applying to general surgery residency. While all the previously described measures may be of some use, members of the surgical community need to think radically out of the box to generate ideas that will entice more US seniors to apply to general surgery. What certainly will not work is nostalgia for the days of "this is how it was in our day." Not only are medical students tired of this, but so are many surgeons. "This is how it was done in our day, and this is how good we were in the past" is not a justification to repeat the errors of the past. The constant theme of how surgeons were so good in the past and how the present students and residents are so bad is definitely not going to attract anyone anymore to surgery. It is highly inappropriate to state that a whole generation of current students are not worthy to be trained as surgeons. It is equally inappropriate to expect utopian, all metric-based perfection in trainees when current surgeons are less than perfect and practice in a world that is equally imperfect. Instead one should learn from the best of the past, avoid the errors of the past, and get acquainted with the millennial and postmillenial generations to identify those talented medical students who will become the surgeons of future. Intelligence and industry are definitely not in dearth in these bright young men and women, but what is needed is the ability to channel that talent respectfully in the right direction to maintain the ranks of surgery.

Surgical Residency

The primary theme at this stage is to encourage more general surgery residents to practice general surgery.

Change perceptions about general surgery

It is not uncommon for general surgery residents in training to say that they want to pursue "just" general surgery. This gives the impression that pursuing general surgery as a career right after training is in some ways inferior or less gratifying than to pursuing a fellowship after completion of residency. The surgical graduate medical education (GME) community needs to encourage those residents who want to enter practice after completion of residency by providing guidance and outlining the rewards of such a career choice.

General surgery is a high-priority specialty

The 21st report[29] published by the Council on Graduate Medical Education (COGME) in August 2013 is titled as: "Improving value in Graduate Medical Education.[1] The report emphasizes the need for obtaining greater value for public funds allocated to GME by redirecting funds to certain high-priority specialties. These high-priority specialties were identified based on several factors including the need for these services in the future. General surgery is 1 of the 6 high-priority specialties identified by COGME for increases in GME funding. The importance of general surgery is being recognized at the federal level and state level, and by elected officials. It would be appropriate to highlight this to surgical residents planning to pursue general surgery so as to enable them to feel satisfied with their career path.

Appraisal of location of surgery residency programs

There were 257 general surgery residency programs included in the match process for 2015, with 1224 available categorical general surgery residency positions.[30] A review of the geographic location of the residency programs reveals significant variability in the number of general surgery residency programs per state (**Table 8**). There are certain states with more than 20 general surgery residency programs, whereas there are some states that have none. This variability could be a reflection of the state's population, which drives the need for surgical services. At the same time, presence of fewer programs or none in some states could explain the difficulty in attracting general surgeons to practice in those states. This could contribute to the uneven distribution of general surgeons across the United States.[5] Attempts should be made to support new programs or expand existing programs in states with low numbers of surgeons to address the lopsided distribution of general surgical workforce across the nation. Similarly, introduction of rural tracks during residency is likely to increase the number of graduates settling in rural areas and practicing general surgery.

Tackling duty hour regulations

The debate on the pros and cons of the duty hour regulations[31] has been vigorous from its inception and is likely to continue unabated. In the interim, several studies have been published about the pros and cons on the effects of the duty hour rules on resident education and patient care. For the purposes of this article, one study published by Philibert and colleagues[32] will be referred to. This study, published in 2013 by the leadership of ACGME, was an attempt to determine the effect of the duty hour rules on resident education, patient safety, and other metrics. Of the 7 studies that reported worse patient safety outcomes, 5 of them included surgical specialties. The duty hour regulations were introduced without any evidence to suggest benefits to resident education or patient care. It is hoped that this question will be answered in the near future by the FIRST (Flexibility In duty hour Requirements for Surgical Training) trial,[33] which was initiated in July 2014; the interim results are eagerly anticipated. In the interim, the surgical community should continue to refine training methods within the confines of restricted duty hours, which in some form are likely to be permanent. This will ensure that surgeons of competence who feel comfortable to go out into practice without feeling the need to pursue additional fellowship training are trained.

Gender-friendly environment in surgical residency

Nearly 47% of students in medical schools across the United States are women, and they also constitute 46% of the resident community.[34] Female surgeons account for

Table 8
Number of general surgery residency programs per state

Number of General Surgery Residency Programs per State			
High Number of Programs per State		Low Number of Programs per State	
New York	26	Kansas	2
Pennsylvania	20	Oklahoma	2
California	18	Nebraska	2
Ohio	14	North Dakota	1
Texas	14	South Dakota	0
Michigan	12	Wyoming	0

15.4% of the general surgery workforce, and they constitute a larger fraction (32%) of the number of residents in general surgical residency programs.[4] The number of women seeking a career in general surgery is likely to increase to mirror the increasing number of female medical students. Surgical leadership should ensure that the environment is conducive to address issues specific to female surgical residents, such as the ability to take maternity leave without adverse consequences. Although professional growth is expected during residency, no one would hope that it comes at the expense of stifling personal growth. The extended leave option and the 6-year option put forth by the American Board of Surgery (ABS) are laudable steps in that direction.[35] Despite these measures, female residents still tend to deliver the news of their pregnancy to the program director with cautious trepidation instead of sharing the news with boundless joy. Further measures such as those instituted by the ABS can entice more female students to apply to general surgery and contribute to the workforce.

Progression during residency based on assessment and testing in written, oral, and technical skills after graduation
The current system assures progression through residency without any testing unless there are serious deficiencies. Although a return to pyramidal system is unwarranted, the ability to test competency in all domains before progression to the next year will ensure that training surgeons of competence are trained. Similarly, the technical skills of graduates are not currently tested. Greater assimilation of simulation will provide the opportunities to test surgical skills. Testing proficiency, not only in written and oral skills, but also technical skills, will ensure that graduates are confident to enter the practice of general surgery without pursuing additional fellowship training.

Shorter training period/absorb training practices from other parts of the world
The 5 year period for training general surgeons in the United States is considered sacrosanct. While the surgical community is accustomed to the 5-year period, there is no evidence to suggest that this is the appropriate period to train general surgeons of competence. It is likely that more time is needed or just as likely that general surgeons could be trained in shorter periods of time. Such a debate would cause much consternation, particularly in the environment of restricted duty hours, which many feel has already compromised general surgical training.

There are several rotations that are currently part of the general surgery residency training curriculum that contribute minimally to the practice of the current general surgeon. This trend may continue to increase as more specialties become highly specialized. Is it possible to envision the general surgeon of the future whose scope of practice consists of treating only the most common general surgical conditions and refer others to the specialists? Is it possible to train the general surgeon of the future who is competent in addressing the most common general surgical conditions only with minimal exposure to other surgical conditions? If such is the case, is it possible that the general surgeon of the future can be trained in a shorter period of time? A shorter training cycle will also provide the malleability needed to address workforce shortages rapidly.

Surgical training systems across the world are of varying duration. It would be beneficial to explore these various systems to provide the stimulus to develop surgical residency programs of shorter or longer duration. The training system in the United States is considered by many to be the model for surgical training. Before one discounts other training systems, however, it would be prudent to recall that Halsted pioneered the residency system based on his observations while traveling abroad.

System should be rapidly adaptable to new diseases and technology
The content of surgical residency training should reflect the patterns of surgical diseases and also the adoption of new technology. One should be nimble to be able to take emphasis away from pathologies such as peptic ulcer disease and be able to focus it on newer procedures such as bariatric surgery. Similarly, one also should be able to assimilate training in newer technologies in a rapid fashion, which can be aided by simulation-based training. Training in new technologies during residency itself will decrease the need for pursuing additional fellowship training just to acquire skills in procedures based on new technology.

Promote global health rotations
The current generation of medical students is passionate about global health.[36] Unless avenues to undertake global health rotations are provided, bright students may choose other specialties that are more open to such opportunities. Residents who undertake such rotations could also be more likely to provide care in underserved areas, which can help address the uneven distribution of surgeons.

Target attrition
It is beyond the scope of this article to review the causes behind attrition during residency.[37] This multifactorial issues need to be tackled so that bright residents can be retained to complete their training and join the surgical workforce.

Lobbying to increase the number of residency positions
The "Training Tomorrow's Doctors Today Act" bill[38] was introduced in 2013 to support 15,000 new residency positions over a 5 year period. It is unlikely that this bill will come to fruition, but the surgical community should continue to lobby to increase the number of residency positions to boost the ranks of the surgical workforce.

In summary, the surgical training system in the United States pioneered by Halsted is considered to be one of the best in the world and has served as a durable model for the United States and many other countries in the world. Although this model has stood the test of time, the health care system in the United States has witnessed significant changes in the recent times. These changes will have a significant bearing on how the future generation of general surgeons is trained, which in turn will have a profound influence on the surgical workforce. Complacency cannot be the order of the day. The surgical community needs to be proactive in initiating/embracing the changes and instituting innovative practices to the surgical training paradigm. This will require radical thinking, which might well go against the conventional wisdom. But unless the approach involves such radical ideas based on the principles of creative destruction, one runs the risk of becoming irrelevant or control of training future surgeons might be ceded to other entities. The history of the field of surgery is punctuated by surgeons who have demonstrated great leadership and made significant contributions to the entire field of graduate medical education. The Halstedian model was indeed pioneered by a surgeon. The time is ripe again for the surgical community to rise to the challenge and modify/develop new surgical training paradigms that can serve as seminal models of graduate medical education. It is hoped that these models will serve the nation just as admirably well as the Halstedian model did in training generations of physicians and surgeons for well over a century.

REFERENCES

1. Council on Medical Education, Hospitals of the American Medical Association. Essential in a hospital approved for residencies in specialties. JAMA 1933;100: 899–910.

2. Definition of workforce, Oxford Dictionaries. Available at: http://www.oxforddictionaries.com/us/definition/american_english/workforce. Accessed June 14, 2015.
3. Bureau of Labor Statistics, occupational outlook handbook, physicians and surgeons. Available at: http://www.bls.gov/ooh/healthcare/physicians-and-surgeons.htm. Accessed June 14, 2015.
4. The surgical workforce in the United States: profile and recent trends. American College of Surgeons Health Policy Research Institute. Available at: http://www.acshpri.org/documents/ACSHPRI_Surgical_Workforce_in_US_apr2010.pdf. Accessed June 14, 2015.
5. Distribution of surgical workforce in the United States, American College of Surgeons Health Policy Institute. Available at: http://www.acshpri.org/documents/SurgeonMaps2006-2011_Oct2012.pdf. Accessed June 21, 2015.
6. Centers for Disease Control and Prevention. FastStats. Available at: http://www.cdc.gov/nchs/fastats/inpatient-surgery.htm. Accessed June 14, 2015.
7. Centers for Disease Control and Prevention. National Hospital Discharge Surgery: 2010 table, Procedures by selected patient characteristics- Number by procedure category and age. Available at: http://www.cdc.gov/nchs/data/nhds/4procedures/2010pro4_numberprocedureage.pdf Accessed June 14, 2015.
8. United States Census Bureau, Population Projections. 2014 National Population Projections: summary tables. Available at: http://www.census.gov/population/projections/data/national/2014/summarytables.html. Accessed June 14, 2015.
9. Valentine RJ, Jones A, Biester TW, et al. General Surgery workloads and practice patterns in the United States, 2007 to 2009. A 10-year update from the American Board of Surgery. Ann Surg 2011;254:520–5.
10. Population profile of the United States, 1997. Available at: https://www.census.gov/prod/3/98pubs/p23-194.pdf. Accessed June 14, 2015.
11. United States Census Bureau, Age and Sex Composition in the United States: 2007. Available at: http://www.census.gov/population/age/data/2007comp.html. Accessed June 14, 2015.
12. NRMP historical reports. Available at: http://www.nrmp.org/match-data/nrmp-historical-reports/. Accessed June 14, 2015.
13. Health Resources and Service Administration. Physician supply and demand: projections to 2020. Available at: http://bhpr.hrsa.gov/healthworkforce/supplydemand/medicine/physician2020projections.pdf. Accessed June 21, 2015.
14. Health Resources and Service Administration. The physician workforce: projections and research into current issues affecting supply and demand. Available at: http://bhpr.hrsa.gov/healthworkforce/reports/physwfissues.pdf. Accessed June 21, 2015.
15. Health Resources and Service Administration. Projecting the supply of nonprimary care specialty and subspecialty clinicians: 2010-2025. Available at: http://bhpr.hrsa.gov/healthworkforce/supplydemand/usworkforce/clinicalspecialties/clinicalspecialties.pdf. Accessed June 21, 2015.
16. National residency matching program, data for the year 1978. Available at: http://www.nrmp.org/wp-content/uploads/2013/08/resultsanddata1984.pdf. Accessed June 27, 2015.
17. National residency matching program, data for the year 2014. Available at: http://www.nrmp.org/wp-content/uploads/2014/04/Main-Match-Results-and-Data-2014.pdf. Accessed June 27, 2015.

18. Are C, Stoddard HA, Northam L, et al. An early exposure in surgical anatomy to provide first-year medical students with an early exposure to general surgery: a pilot study. J Surg Educ 2009;66:186–9.

19. Are C, Stoddard HA, Thompson JS, et al. The influence of surgical demonstrations during an anatomy course on the perceptions of first-year medical students towards surgeons and a surgical career. J Surg Educ 2010;67: 320–4.

20. Patel MS, Mowlds DS, Khalsa B, et al. Early intervention to promote medical students interest in surgery and surgical subspecialties. J Surg Educ 2013;70: 81–6.

21. Haggerty KA, Beaty CA, George TJ, et al. Increased exposure improves recruitment: early results of a program designed to attract medical students into surgical careers. Ann Thorac Surg 2014;97:2111–4.

22. Kozar RA, Anderson KD, Escobar-Chaves SL, et al. Preclinical students: who are surgeons? J Surg Res 2004;15:113–6.

23. Stone JP, Charette JH, McPhalen DF, et al. Under the knife: Medical student perception of intimidation and mistreatment. J Surg Educ 2015;72:749–53.

24. Quillin RC 3rd, Pritts TA, Davis BR, et al. Surgeons underestimate their influence on medical students entering surgery. J Surg Res 2012;177:201–6.

25. Are C, Stoddard HA, O' Holleran B, et al. A multinational perspective on lifestyle and other perceptions of contemporary medical students about general surgery. Ann Surg 2012;256:378–86.

26. Rollman BL, Mead LA, Wang NY, et al. Medical specialty and the incidence of divorce. N Engl J Med 1997;336:800–3.

27. Ly DP, Seabury SA, Jena AB. Divorce among physicians and other healthcare professionals in the United States: analysis of census survey data. BMJ 2015; 350:h706.

28. Harms BA, Heise CP, Gould JC, et al. A 25- year single institution analysis of health, practice and fate of general surgeons. Ann Surg 2005;242:520–6.

29. Council on Graduate Medical Education. Twenty-first report. Improving value in Graduate Medical Education. 2013. Available at: http://www.hrsa.gov/advisorycommittees/bhpradvisory/cogme/Reports/twentyfirstreport.pdf. Accessed June 27, 2015.

30. National residency matching program, results and data 2015 main residency match. Available at: http://www.nrmp.org/wp-content/uploads/2015/05/Main-Match-Results-and-Data-2015_final.pdf. Accessed June 27, 2015.

31. Accreditation Council on Graduate Medical Education. Resident duty hours in the learning and working environment. Comparison of 2003 and 2011 standards. Available at: https://www.acgme.org/acgmeweb/Portals/0/PDFs/dh-ComparisonTable2003v2011.pdf. Accessed June 27, 2015.

32. Philibert I, Nasca T, Brigham T, et al. Duty-hour limits and patient care and resident outcomes: can high-quality studies offer insights into complex relationships? Annu Rev Med 2013;64:467–83.

33. Flexibility in duty hour requirements for surgical trainees trial. Available at: http://www.thefirsttrial.org/. Accessed June 27, 2015.

34. The state of women in academic medicine: the pipeline and pathways to leadership, 2013-2014. Association of American Medical Colleges. Available at: https://www.acgme.org/acgmeweb/Portals/0/PDFs/dh-ComparisonTable2003v2011.pdf. Accessed June 27, 2015.

35. Leave policy. American Board of Surgery. Available at: http://www.absurgery.org/default.jsp?policygsleave. Accessed June 27, 2015.

36. Powell AC, Casey K, Liewehr DJ, et al. Results of a national survey of surgical resident interest in international experience, elective and volunteerism. J Am Coll Surg 2009;208:304–12.
37. Gifford E, Galante J, Kaji AJ, et al. Factors associated with general surgery residents' desire to leave residency programs: a multi-institutional study. JAMA Surg 2014;149:948–53.
38. "Training Tomorrow's Doctors Today Act." Available at: https://www.aamc.org/ newsroom/newsreleases/330948/031413.html. Accessed June 28, 2015.

Education and Training to Address Specific Needs During the Career Progression of Surgeons

CrossMark

Ajit K. Sachdeva, MD, FRCSC*, Patrice Gabler Blair, MPH,
Linda K. Lupi, MBA

KEYWORDS

- Lifelong learning in surgery • Entry into surgical practice • Development of expertise
- Skills in new procedures and technologies • Reentry into surgical practice
- Mentoring, preceptoring, coaching, proctoring
- Professional activities in late surgical careers • Education and training

KEY POINTS

- The education and training needs of practicing surgeons continue to evolve in the changing health care environment.
- New and innovative education and training methods that are based on contemporary practice-based learning and improvement, and continuous professional development methods are needed to support surgeons during transitions and throughout various phases of their professional careers.
- Cutting-edge technologies, blended models, simulation, mentoring, preceptoring, and integrated education and training approaches can be designed to meet surgeon-specific needs and play critical roles in helping surgeons maintain lifelong practices of providing the best surgical care.

BACKGROUND

Monumental changes continue to impact surgical practice and health care in general. Sharp focus on outcomes of care, value, and accountability; major emphasis on improving quality of care and ensuring patient safety; impact of new regulations;

Disclosure Statement: The authors of the article, "Education and Training to Address Specific Needs During the Career Progression of Surgeons" affirm that they have no commercial or financial conflicts of interest. Also, there were no funding sources that supported this work.
Disclaimer: The opinions expressed in this article are those of the authors and do not necessarily represent the official position of the American College of Surgeons.
Division of Education, American College of Surgeons, 633 North Saint Clair Street, Chicago, IL 60611, USA
* Corresponding author.
E-mail address: asachdeva@facs.org

and evolving patient expectations are all affecting the practices of surgeons. These changes are also increasing stress in the professional lives of surgeons who need to constantly balance various priorities to provide the best care to patients. Innovative surgical education and training can be of immense value in addressing many mandates and challenges, and are essential to delivering surgical care of the highest quality.

The continuum of professional development during the career progression of surgeons needs to be considered as new education and training methods are developed and implemented. During residency training, and before that in medical school, structured systems exist to offer individuals specific learning opportunities that are linked to defined curricula and specific milestones that support advancement from one level to the next. The recent emphasis on transitions from medical school to surgery residency, during the years of surgical training, and from residency training to practice has resulted in the identification of a variety of challenges that need to be addressed against the backdrop of the rapidly changing learning environment and new regulations. The major focus on the education and training of medical students and surgical trainees is in sharp contrast to the relatively limited attention that has been devoted to the continuing education and training of surgeons during different phases in their professional careers. This is indeed paradoxical, because time spent in medical school and in specialty or subspecialty training is relatively short in comparison with the decades spent in surgical practice. The challenges during these latter years are unique because transformational changes in health care and new regulatory mandates continue to impact surgical practices directly, and because individual practices vary immensely. In addition, there is no structured curriculum to guide practicing surgeons in their lifelong learning pursuits. A number of practical limitations impact the participation of surgeons in education and training as well. Taking time away from busy practices and arranging appropriate coverage for patients during the period of absence can present formidable challenges. Also, the additional expenses associated with participation in cutting-edge education and training programs can deter surgeons from participating in these programs.

Advances in continuing medical education (CME) have lagged behind those in medical student education and residency training despite the potential for major positive impact of education and training on patient care during the long periods of time surgeons are actively engaged in practice. For approximately 20 years, concerns have consistently been expressed about the effectiveness of traditional CME in improving the performance of physicians and health care outcomes.[1–4] Some progress has been made in designing, testing, and implementing new methods to increase the effectiveness of CME. These methods have included learner-centered approaches, interactive sessions, sequenced programs that involve multiple sessions to achieve specific goals, audits of practice and feedback, and support from local opinion leaders.[2,3] These methods continue to be introduced into CME activities, but there is still great opportunity for major innovation.

THE NEW PARADIGM OF CONTINUOUS PROFESSIONAL DEVELOPMENT AND PRACTICE-BASED LEARNING AND IMPROVEMENT

An entirely new paradigm of continuous professional development (CPD) has been proposed to replace the conventional CME model.[5] CPD includes several distinct characteristics. It focuses on lifelong learning that is based on needs of individuals as opposed to needs of large learner groups, and involves the use of a range of learner-driven and learner-centered education and training methods. CPD is offered in venues that extend beyond traditional lecture halls and conference rooms, and uses a variety of learning formats and blended methods to achieve optimal results. Clinical practice locations and simulated environments are well suited to the delivery of CPD. Also, CPD is more comprehensive in scope than traditional CME, and can be used to address not just the clinical domain but also practice management, leadership, teamwork, administration, and a host of other professional activities.

Another important approach that needs to be used to offer practicing surgeons effective education and training involves the use of practice-based learning and improvement (PBLI).[5,6] Approximately 15 years ago, 6 core competencies, including PBLI, were defined by the Accreditation Council for Graduate Medical Education and the American Board of Medical Specialties, and since then all trainees and practicing physicians have been required to acquire and demonstrate these competencies throughout their careers. Many standards of certifying and accrediting bodies are based on the core competencies. A number of special strategies need to be considered with regard to addressing the core competencies. Different levels of emphasis need to be placed on individual core competencies during various phases in the careers of physicians. Also, the core competencies are used in combination by physicians to provide care to patients; thus, they must be taught and learned in an integrated fashion. For practicing surgeons, PBLI should be considered central in education and training efforts. It helps to identify and define learning needs within all other competencies and can also be very helpful in addressing those needs. The PBLI Cycle includes 4 steps: (1) identifying areas for improvement ideally through data-driven, systematic gap analyses and robust metacognitive processes; (2) engagement in learning through participation in programs and activities that are based on effective CPD approaches; (3) application of new knowledge and skills to practice, facilitated by involvement of mentors, preceptors, and proctors and support from local experts; and (4) checking for improvement, using data when possible. These 4 steps of the PBLI Cycle should be repeated to help physicians reach the highest levels of performance based on their aptitude and internal motivation. Continuing education and training for surgeons should be anchored to the PBLI Cycle and based on contemporary CPD methods. Continuing education and training also need to be aimed at ongoing improvement over the lifetime of professional practice, and specific goals along this journey should serve as milestones only, and not be considered definitive end points.

A major motivator for practicing surgeons that encourages them to participate in education and training programs is achievement of specific goals at different steps during the lifelong journey toward expertise, which may progress to mastery. This dynamic progression underscores the need for frequent formative and summative assessments that should be built into education and training programs and coupled with specific feedback to improve performance. Courses focusing on cognitive skills and judgment should include pre-tests and post-tests that are anchored to specific learning objectives. Skills courses need to include objective verification of skills by expert faculty or through use of appropriate simulators. Although ongoing formative and summative assessments that are part of CPD activities are aimed at continual improvement and do not lead to formal pass/fail decisions, these assessments must be valid and reliable for the results to be credible and for learners to receive useful data that will catalyze positive change. Objective verification of knowledge and skills and benchmarking of the results with national, regional, and local standards are critical steps in the process of validation of knowledge and skills. Data from robust assessments also can be used during the process of credentialing and granting privileges, and should be helpful to surgeons in their efforts to earn new privileges and maintain existing privileges. Assessment data also affirm achievement of specific milestones and give surgeons a sense of accomplishment, which instills joy in the learning process.

FOCUS ON MAINTENANCE OF CERTIFICATION AND MAINTENANCE OF LICENSURE

The requirements for Maintenance of Certification (MOC) and the concept of Maintenance of Licensure (MOL) continue to evolve.[7,8] Current MOC Standards include the following 4 parts: Professionalism and Professional Standing; Lifelong Learning and Self-Assessment; Assessment of Knowledge, Judgment, and Skills; and Improvement in Medical Practice.[7] Parts 2 and 4 of MOC can be viewed as linked and interdependent, and should be considered together for purposes of education and training. Collection of data from practice outcomes and analyses of practices needed to fulfill requirements of Part 4 of MOC should help in defining education and training needs that may be addressed through participation in appropriate programs, which would then fulfill the requirements of Part 2 of MOC. Also, if the requirements of Part 2 are adequately addressed, they should result in a positive impact on practices, as measured through MOC Part 4 activities. Various certifying boards have specific requirements for self-assessment credits as well. For example, the American Board of Surgery requires that at least 60 of the 90 CME credits during the 3-year MOC cycle must include self-assessment and that each surgeon must achieve at least 75% on tests to be granted self-assessment credits.[9] The MOL framework includes 3 core components: reflective self-assessment; assessment of knowledge and skills; and performance in practice.[8] The MOL components are similar to the parts of MOC and activities used to fulfill MOC requirements may be relevant for MOL as well. The MOL framework was approved by the Federation of State Medical Boards in 2010, and a few states are currently conducting pilot programs.[8] In addition, individual state medical boards have specific requirements for licensure. For example, some states require CME credits in special topics, such as patient safety, risk management, ethics, pain management, palliative care, and end-of-life care.[10]

A major goal of CPD and PBLI activities should be to help surgeons meet various regulatory mandates, including those relating to MOC and MOL. National professional organizations and academic medical centers continue to offer a range of education and training programs to help surgeons fulfill MOC requirements. The American College of Surgeons (ACS) Division of Education offers a vast array of standard-setting continuing education and training programs that can help practicing surgeons in fulfilling MOC requirements and staying current with the latest advances in surgery and related fields. These programs include the transformed Annual Clinical Congress that offers a broad range of educational programs, including scientific presentations, panel presentations, didactic courses, surgical skills courses, multimedia programs, and small group activities. Special certificates are provided to participants to address MOC and licensure requirements as well as other regulatory mandates, and to support credentialing and privileging. The renowned and evidence-based *Surgical Education and Self-Assessment Program (SESAP)* is offered in various formats to support individual goals and learning styles, and remains the premier self-assessment program for surgeons. This program includes a unique guided learning model that is, aimed at enhancing cognitive skills. The evidence-based *Selected Readings in General Surgery* includes syntheses of the current literature and topical reviews of surgical content. This program provides comprehensive coverage of the topics in a cyclical fashion and is offered in various formats. The Comprehensive General Surgery Review Course and the shorter Review Course at the Clinical

Congress cover the breadth of General Surgery content. The impact of these programs and other offerings of the ACS Division of Education extends well beyond the regulatory requirements and mandates. Many of these programs include self-assessment models that require a score higher than 75% and some programs require a perfect score of 100% to earn self-assessment credits. The perfect score can be achieved through re-review of specific content, guided learning, and multiple attempts at taking the test. These learning and testing models require active participation of the learner, and involve repetition and reinforcement, which contribute to the achievement of expertise. The aforementioned programs also support efforts of surgeons to stay on the cutting-edge of their professional activities and motivate surgeons to pursue higher goals.

FOCUS ON CRITICAL TRANSITIONS DURING THE CAREER PROGRESSION OF PRACTICING SURGEONS

Across the decades of professional work, knowledge and skills continually evolve and surgeons go through many transitions, several of which are critical. These transitions present major challenges to the surgeons and offer great opportunities for significant impact through innovative education and training. The critical phases during the career progression of practicing surgeons are as follows: entry into practice, which includes the initial 2 to 3 years when individuals settle into their new careers; the core period of professional practice that can span 20 to 30 years or even longer periods, when individuals continually refine existing skills, acquire new skills, and strive toward achievement of expertise; and the later years, which generally encompass the last 3 to 5 years of professional careers before retirement, when surgeons begin to wind down their clinical practices and often turn to other professional endeavors. Each of these phases has its own unique needs that must be addressed through specific education and training strategies and methods. A comprehensive approach that spans the continuum of surgical careers should help in keeping surgeons actively engaged and excited about their skills and contributions, and benefit patients, colleagues, surgical trainees, other health professionals, the surgical profession, and society at large.

The model used by the ACS Division of Education to focus on the career progression of surgeons involves specific focus on critical transitions that may result in vulnerabilities and offer opportunities for maximal impact. This is illustrated in **Fig. 1.**

Entry into Practice

Entry into surgical practice has always been a major transition in the career progression of individuals, and has recently received significant attention as readiness of

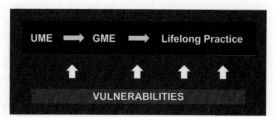

Fig. 1. Focus on the career progression of surgeons with special attention to key transitions from undergraduate medical education (UME) to graduate medical education (GME) and throughout lifelong practice.

surgery residents for practice has been questioned.[11] Deficiencies in clinical, technical, and practice management skills have been cited by a variety of individuals receiving junior surgeons who have recently completed training. Worries have also been expressed about the confidence of the junior surgeons to perform certain procedures. An interesting finding is that the perceptions of junior surgeons entering surgical practice regarding their skills and readiness for practice are different from the perceptions of those accepting these individuals. These differences need to be bridged to ensure smooth entry of junior surgeons into practice settings.

In 2012, the ACS Division of Education partnered with the Accreditation Council for Graduate Medical Education to convene a national invitational conference to define key issues relating to transition to practice in surgery and to propose solutions to address the challenges identified. Several recommendations focused on residency training and addressed redesign of the surgery residency training model, interventions aimed at chief residents to prepare them for independent practice, and evaluation and verification of knowledge and skills of residents before graduation. Recommendations also focused on the initial period of entry into surgical practice and addressed evaluation and verification of knowledge and skills of individuals entering practice; mentoring, preceptoring, and proctoring of individuals entering practice; use of new technologies, including telementoring, telepreceptoring, and teleproctoring to support individuals entering practice; and strategies to address a variety of regulatory and legal issues, specifically those pertaining to credentialing and privileging.[11]

Assessment of an entering junior surgeon needs to be conducted within the context of the specific practice environment in which the individual will practice, and should include a sign-off process attesting to the proficiency of the individual. Mentoring and preceptoring should be offered routinely to the junior surgeon and specific steps taken to address any gaps identified. Simulation can be used to assess skills, remediate as needed, and offer the junior surgeon opportunities to practice and improve his or her skills in safe environments. Mentoring should be offered routinely, and considered supportive rather than punitive. The mentor can be of great help in building on the strengths of the junior surgeon, identifying and addressing specific needs, supporting the junior surgeon as he or she navigates various complex situations in the practice environment, and serving as an advocate for the junior surgeon. Mentorship involves a comprehensive and intense, long-term professional relationship that can have profound positive effects on both the mentor and the protégé.[12] This relationship is multidimensional and is based on the developmental-contextual framework. The length of the mentorship should be specifically tailored to the needs of the junior surgeon and the characteristics of the practice environment. In certain situations, mentoring may need to be provided by several individuals rather than a single person, based on the needs of the junior surgeon. Preceptorship also can be helpful to the junior surgeon. This is a short-term professional relationship between a preceptee and an expert in the field, who serves as the preceptor and helps the preceptee acquire specific skills. Also, a proctor may be assigned to formally assess the knowledge and skills of the entering junior surgeon through direct observations of the junior surgeon's performance and review of patient care outcomes. The roles and responsibilities of a proctor are very different from those of a preceptor, and the principal responsibility of a proctor is to share the findings of the assessments with the chief of surgery or the institutional credentialing and privileging committee.[13] Assessment information from the proctor and data from patient care outcomes can be used to address the requirements of Focused Professional Practice Evaluation and Ongoing Professional Practice Evaluation requirements, as defined by The Joint Commission.[14]

The use of new technologies can help with education, training, and assessment efforts and support the on-boarding of junior surgeons. The junior surgeons entering practice may need support and guidance from their senior colleagues and other experts for the first few years after they have entered practice, especially if they encounter a difficult surgical challenge or an infrequent problem. With appropriate experience, mentorship, and preceptorship, such needs should diminish over time.

The ACS Division of Education is currently developing guidelines with regard to on-boarding of junior surgeons entering practice. Efforts are also under way to design and test new models to support this transition, and to disseminate information on best practices from the different environments of surgical care. New methods for workplace and simulation-based assessments are also being designed, which would be helpful in assessing the skills of the junior surgeons entering practice and addressing any gaps that are identified.

The Core Period of Professional Practice

During the several decades of the core period of surgical practice, surgeons need to continually refine their skills, acquire new skills, and achieve and maintain expertise. The PBLI Cycle and contemporary CPD methods previously outlined in this article remain pivotal throughout this period in the career progression of surgeons. Ongoing refinement of skills requires objective assessments of performance and outcomes, specific feedback, reflection by the learner, and sufficient practice in real and simulated environments. Benchmarking with metrics relating to expert performance and external standards, when available, is helpful in this context. Review of videotapes of an operation with an expert can be of value in refining surgical technique and intraoperative judgment.[15] Mentoring and preceptoring previously described in this article can be very helpful in maintaining and enhancing skills. Coaching has recently received considerable attention as an effective mechanism to refine existing skills. Three elements of coaching have been described. These include setting goals, encouraging and motivating, and developing and guiding.[16] A comprehensive surgical coaching model recently published in the literature includes objective assessment, structured debriefing, feedback, behavior modeling, and guided self-reflection.[17] Barriers to coaching surgeons in practice include a lack of recognition of the need for technical improvement, concern about appearing incompetent, and worry about losing autonomy.[18] For coaching to be widely accepted, a major national effort will need to be launched to change the culture within surgery and other health care professions, so that coaching activities do not carry a stigma and are considered routine in efforts to continually refine skills and achieve higher levels of performance. Professional societies, such as the ACS, could play a vital role in this regard.

Development and maintenance of expertise leading to mastery in surgery are also important during the core period of professional practice and require deliberate practice coupled with specific and timely feedback.[19] Discussions regarding achievement of expertise have often focused on the number of hours of practice; however, the critical element in developing expertise is ongoing establishment of goals that exceed current level of performance and drive the learner toward higher levels of excellence. The process of achieving expertise and mastery can be readily supported through simulation-based training. The standardized and controlled simulation environments provide excellent opportunities for deliberate practice and allow learners to stretch up to and beyond the limits of their competence and confidence without placing patients at risk. Also, individuals can learn prevention of errors and recovery from errors without harm to patients. Mentoring, coaching, and simulation-based training, in combination should be helpful in promoting expertise and mastery in surgery throughout the core period of practice.

Another effective tool to enhance performance and outcomes, support development of expertise and mastery, and address all core competencies in an integrated fashion is the Surgery Morbidity and Mortality (M + M) Conference. This conference has served both quality improvement and educational functions for many generations and remains central to the educational efforts within surgery departments. The peer feedback and support in the M + M Conference can be of immense help in improving performance. Certain strategies can be used to realize the full educational and quality improvement potential of the M + M Conference. These include adequate preparation before the conference, effective organization of the conference, selection of a moderator who is a skilled surgeon and well respected by peers, appropriate synthesis of the discussions, clear articulation of conclusions, and planned follow-up. Excessive emphasis on systems of care stemming from efforts to improve patient safety has, at times, led to insufficient emphasis on the performance and responsibilities of individuals and teams. An appropriate balance between these areas of focus is needed.[20] Recent enhancements in the design and implementation of M + M Conferences have improved the value of this conference. Such efforts should continue to keep the M + M Conference at the center of quality improvement and educational efforts.

Advances in science and technology continue to significantly impact surgical practice. Surgeons need to continually strive to assess evolving practice needs and pursue acquisition of skills in new procedures and technologies to provide the best care to patients. An important first step is to thoroughly evaluate the new procedure or technology to determine its relevance to the surgeon's practice. Evidence relating to the efficiency and effectiveness of the new procedure or technology must be evaluated carefully. Also, the practice patterns of the surgeon, needs of the patients served, and the local resources available need to be considered.[13] If a decision is made to adopt a new procedure or new technology in the surgeon's practice, the surgeon must participate in a comprehensive and multistep training program. Established principles of skills training should be used to design and implement effective training programs for surgeons. The key principles are as follows. Mastery-based learning techniques should be used to help individuals achieve preestablished standards and specific goals and objectives. Deliberate practice and specific feedback need to be essential components of the training model. Distributed training that permits phased acquisition of the skills over a period of time has been demonstrated to be more effective with regard to retention and transfer of the technical skills as compared with massed training that is offered in a concentrated fashion over a short period of time.[21] Simulations and simulators can be very helpful within the context of acquiring new skills. Simulation-based training allows deliberate practice in safe settings using standardized training models. A major shortcoming of many skills training programs is insufficient focus on the safe transfer of the newly acquired skills from the training environment to the operating room. This requires structured preceptoring.[12,22] Several models of preceptorship have been attempted; however, practical limitations, regulatory challenges, and risks of liability have prevented their widespread adoption. National efforts through the leadership of professional organizations like the ACS are needed to address these major challenges. The outcomes of the surgeon with regard to the new procedure or technology must be monitored for a period of time following the preceptorship and steps taken to address any gaps that are identified. Periodic reinforcement of the newly acquired skills is also necessary to prevent decrement of these skills.

A number of recent advances have been made with regard to preceptoring and monitoring of outcomes following skills training, to support safe and effective introduction of new procedures into practice. An innovative multistep model that involves participation in courses followed by supervised operating under the preceptorship of experts has been designed to train established colorectal surgeons across England in performing laparoscopic colorectal surgery. These preceptors sign-off on the skills of the learner surgeons following structured assessments and audits of independent practices.[23,24] In view of the challenges associated with dissemination of this model on a larger scale in the United States, support of the learner surgeons through telepreceptoring is being explored. Such innovative efforts need to be developed further and tested in different surgical settings to make structured preceptoring a reality and to ensure delivery of safe care to patients.

Robust credentialing and privileging processes are key to ensuring patient safety. Principles of surgical privileging and credentialing have been articulated by a Study Group of the American Surgical Association (ASA) and include criteria for granting new surgical privileges. The ASA Study Group recommended that such privileges should be granted based on new education and training and demonstration of technical proficiency in a proctored training environment, with post-privileging review of practice experience in the new procedure for an appropriate interval.[25] These recommendations and information from successful experiences in the field need to be used to create robust processes for credentialing and privileging at various institutions.

Another challenge that surgeons may face during their years in practice is the need to change the focus of their practices or to reenter clinical practice following a period of absence for professional or personal reasons. The practices of surgeons generally become more narrow in scope with time; thus, special steps need to be taken to refresh their skills relating to conditions they have not managed or operations they have not performed recently. Ongoing maintenance of skills through simulation-based retraining or work with a surgeon who possesses expertise in specific conditions or operations can be helpful; however, if the surgeon has had little or no experience with conditions or operations for a period of time, formal preceptorship may be necessary. The issues are similar if surgeons need to reenter practice after a period of absence from clinical work. The American Board of Surgery requires individuals to go through a reentry pathway if they are away from surgical practice for 2 or more years.[26] This pathway needs to include a proctoring plan and outcomes assessment. Other national organizations have also outlined mechanisms for physicians to reenter practice.[27] A finite period of structured preceptorship should be very helpful to surgeons in changing the focus of their practices or reentering practice. The ideal model involves the learner surgeon serving as a preceptee and working with an experienced preceptor at the preceptor's practice location for a period of time. The preceptor should then monitor the performance and outcomes of the preceptee and provide further guidance once the preceptee returns to his or her home institution. A variety of challenges make this model difficult to implement widely.

In recent years, special emphasis has been placed on leadership development within the context of evolving health care systems and the new challenges surgeons face. Leadership training can help surgeons succeed in major leadership positions within surgery departments and institutions. In addition, effective teamwork is considered essential in efforts to promote patient safety and structured teamwork training for surgical teams has been offered at institutions across the country. Many teamwork training courses are based on experiences from other professions and industries. Leadership and team training need to be integral to CPD efforts directed at surgeons. Structured training of operating room teams has demonstrated improvements in risk-adjusted mortality and other quality improvement measures, and has been shown to result in a positive impact on operating room communication and first case starts.[28,29]

The ACS Division of Education has been pursuing many innovative strategies to address the needs of practicing surgeons as they progress through their careers spanning several decades. Transitions during these years have remained an area of special focus. Efforts have been specifically directed at offering programs to refine existing skills, develop and maintain expertise, acquire new skills, and address needs during changes in practices or reentry into practice.

In addition to the programs previously mentioned within the context of addressing MOC requirements and promoting excellence, the ACS Division of Education has been engaged in designing and offering a variety of new skills courses, both at the Annual Clinical Congress and at regional sites. The goal of these efforts is to help surgeons acquire new skills and to refine existing skills, leading to expertise and mastery. A 5-Level Verification Model developed by the Division of Education has been used to assess the new skills of course participants at the completion of training and to provide them with specific certificates based on the verification levels achieved.[22] The 5 levels are as follows: Verification of Attendance; Verification of Satisfactory Completion of Course Objectives; Verification of Knowledge and Skills; Verification of Preceptorial Experience; and Demonstration of Satisfactory Patient Outcomes. These certificates should be helpful during the processes of credentialing and privileging. A new model to validate expertise in surgical skills is currently being designed by the ACS Division of Education.

The goal of creating a national network of state-of-the-art simulation facilities across the country to offer surgeons and surgical teams opportunities to acquire new skills, refine existing skills, and acquire and maintain expertise, led to the ACS Division of Education designing, pilot-testing, and launching a national program to accredit simulation centers in 2005.[30] The accredited simulation centers are called ACS-accredited Education Institutes, and each is accredited as a Comprehensive Institute (Level I) or as a Focused Institute (Level II) based on stringent standards and criteria. Currently there are 89 ACS-accredited Education Institutes located mostly across the United States, with a few abroad. The ACS-accredited Education Institutes are multidisciplinary and aim to foster collaboration across the surgical specialties and among professionals from different fields. The ACS-accredited Education Institutes are also pursuing efforts to offer preceptoring and proctoring, and to support credentialing of surgeons and surgical teams. The ACS-accredited Education Institutes are uniquely positioned to offer opportunities for retraining and reentry to the surgical workforce. These institutes are pursuing high-impact research and development. They remain at the nexus of quality improvement and education and training endeavors at their respective institutions, and are beginning to demonstrate the added value of simulation-based surgical education and training within the new models of health care. A consortium of the ACS-accredited Education Institutes has been created to promote collaboration across these institutions and to share best practices.

The ACS Division of Education has also pursued initiatives to harness a variety of other opportunities. The Surgeons as Leaders Course, now in its 12th year, focuses on the new models of leadership needed for success in the evolving health care environment, and is designed to enhance leadership skills to address a variety of challenges and opportunities, as well as to catalyze culture change. A committee on nontechnical skills was recently appointed to build on the successful experience with nontechnical skills courses at the Annual Clinical Congress, to address fully the needs of surgeons and surgical teams through the design and implementation of new programs. Also, a new committee has been appointed to design models for short-term preceptoring at selected locations, and pilot programs are underway at 2 institutions. A state-of-the-art distance education program offers surgeons and members of surgical teams opportunities to access educational programs at or close to their practice locations. This program also permits design and implementation of innovative blended learning programs.

An integrated approach has been used by the ACS Division of Education to offer cutting-edge education and training programs to surgeons and to increase access to these programs. Certain programs are offered at the Annual Clinical Congress, some are offered at ACS-accredited Education Institutes, and others are made available at practice locations through distance education activities. Blended learning approaches allow surgeons to avail of e-learning programs at their practice locations, take pre-tests, and then come to the Clinical Congress or to an ACS-accredited Education Institute to participate in specific education and training programs. Also, following participation in courses, post-tests and additional learning modules are sent out electronically to the participants. Efforts are underway to link skills courses offered at the Annual Clinical Congress with preceptoring and follow-up at the ACS-accredited Education Institutes, and to link programs of the ACS-accredited Education Institutes with those of the Clinical Congress. This should facilitate participation by the practicing surgeons and increase access to programs. The integrated model for delivery of education and training is depicted in **Fig. 2**.

Professional Activities During the Later Years

During the later years in the professional careers of surgeons, as they start winding down their clinical practices or discontinue certain clinical activities, there is tremendous opportunity to engage these experienced individuals in a variety of education and teaching endeavors. These senior surgeons can be readily engaged in providing clinical care and contributing to teaching in certain settings, such as clinics. They can also teach, demonstrate, and role-model effective professionalism and communication skills at the patient's bedside. If they remain current with the latest advances, they can participate in small group discussions on specific surgical topics with other surgeons, surgery residents, and medical students.

The senior surgeons can provide invaluable leadership for innovative programs focusing on cognitive skills, judgment, and evidence-based surgery. They can also play a vital role in the training activities at simulation centers, assess skills, provide

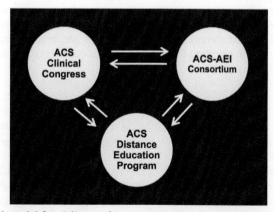

Fig. 2. Integrated model for delivery of innovative ACS education and training.

feedback to the learners, and share assessment results with the appropriate departmental leaders. Some of the senior surgeons who have recently stepped aside from active surgical practice can serve as mentors, preceptors, or coaches for other surgeons and surgical trainees. The mentoring, preceptoring, coaching, and educational skills of the senior surgeons could be enhanced further through targeted faculty development interventions, including special education and training programs. They could also be offered opportunities to participate in other educational activities to keep them current with the latest advances in surgery.

Several institutions across the country have benefited from keeping the senior surgeons involved in their education and training activities. Also, professional societies are offering opportunities to senior surgeons to participate in specific education and training programs. The Thoracic Surgery Directors Association has recruited senior surgeons to teach in their boot camp for entering residents.[31] This has been a very successful endeavor, and has been beneficial to the residents and stimulating for the senior surgeons.

The ACS Division of Education has recruited senior surgeons to lead a variety of innovative educational programs along the lines outlined previously. In addition, several ACS-accredited Education Institutes have engaged senior surgeons in their training activities. A new committee was recently appointed by the ACS Division of Education to fully explore the potential of engaging senior surgeons in education and training activities, offer senior surgeons programs to enhance educational skills as needed, and create national models that would facilitate their participation in these professional endeavors.

SUMMARY

The environment of health care and surgical practice continues to evolve dramatically. Surgeons in practice face many challenges throughout their careers. They have specific needs as they enter practice, throughout the core period of active practice, and then as they wind down their clinical work before retirement. These specific transitions and the career progression process present numerous opportunities to offer innovative education and training. The programs must be founded on sound principles and advances in the science and practice of contemporary surgical education and training. Cutting-edge methods and technologies should be used in blended models to achieve optimal outcomes. In recent years, simulation has been found to be very useful in achieving major education and training goals. The ACS Division of Education continues to address specific needs of surgeons and surgical teams across various phases of their professional careers and is using innovative methods to achieve the best outcomes. Such education and training efforts are essential to providing the best surgical care and supporting the aspirations and career goals of surgeons during various phases in their careers.

REFERENCES

1. Davis DA, Thomson MA, Oxman A, et al. Changing physician performance: a systematic review of the effect of continuing medical education strategies. JAMA 1995;274(9):700–5.
2. Davis D, O'Brien M, Freemantle N, et al. Impact of formal continuing medical education: do conferences, workshops, rounds, and other traditional continuing education activities change physician behavior or health care outcomes? JAMA 1999;282(9):867–74.

3. Mazmanian PE, Davis DA. Continuing medical education and the physician as a learner: guide to the evidence. JAMA 2002;288(9):1057–60.
4. Nissen SE. Reforming the continuing medical education system. JAMA 2015; 313(18):1813–4.
5. Sachdeva AK. The new paradigm of continuing education in surgery. Arch Surg 2005;140(3):264–9.
6. Sachdeva AK, Blair PG. Educating surgery residents in patient safety. Surg Clin North Am 2004;84(6):1669–98.
7. American Board of Medical Specialties. Standards for the ABMS program for Maintenance of Certification (MOC): for implementation in January 2015. Available at: http://www.abms.org/media/1109/standards-for-the-abms-program-for-moc-final.pdf. Accessed September 12, 2015.
8. Federation of State Medical Boards. Maintenance of licensure: fast facts. Available at: https://www.fsmb.org/Media/Default/PDF/FSMB/Foundation/mol-fast-facts.pdf. Accessed September 12, 2015.
9. American Board of Surgery. Maintenance of Certification program. Available at: http://www.absurgery.org/xfer/MOC_Summary.pdf. Accessed September 13, 2015.
10. American College of Surgeons. CME state requirements. Available at: https://www.facs.org/~/media/files/education/cmestatereqmar2015.ashx. Accessed September 13, 2015.
11. Sachdeva AK, Flynn TC, Brigham TP, et al. Interventions to address challenges associated with the transition from residency training to independent surgical practice. Surgery 2014;155(5):867–82.
12. Sachdeva AK. Preceptorship, mentorship, and the adult learner in medical and health sciences education. J Cancer Educ 1996;11(3):131–6.
13. Sachdeva AK, Russell TR. Safe introduction of new procedures and emerging technologies in surgery: education, credentialing, and privileging. Surg Clin North Am 2007;87(4):853–66.
14. Hill S, Herringer J. The Joint Commission. Standards and national patient safety goals: what's new for critical access hospitals in 2012. Available at: http://www.jointcommission.org/assets/1/18/January_12_2012_CAH_Teleconference_final.pdf. Accessed September 13, 2015.
15. Hu YY, Peyre SE, Arriaga AF, et al. Postgame analysis: using video-based coaching for continuous professional development. J Am Coll Surg 2012;214(1): 115–24.
16. Greenberg CC, Ghousseini HN, Pavuluri Quamme SR, et al. Surgical coaching for individual performance improvement. Ann Surg 2015;261(1):32–4.
17. Bonrath EM, Dedy NJ, Gordon LE, et al. Comprehensive surgical coaching enhances surgical skill in the operating room: a randomized controlled trial. Ann Surg 2015;262(2):205–12.
18. Mutabzic D, Mylopoulos M, Murnaghan ML, et al. Coaching surgeons: is culture limiting our ability to improve? Ann Surg 2015;262(2):213–6.
19. Ericsson KA. Deliberate practice and the acquisition and maintenance of expert performance in medicine and related domains. Acad Med 2004;79(10 Suppl): S70–81.
20. Russell JC. Improving surgery: the surgery morbidity and mortality conference. Pharos Alpha Omega Alpha Honor Med Soc 2013;76(3):28–31.
21. Moulton CE, Dubrowski A, MacRae H, et al. Teaching surgical skills: what kind of practice makes perfect? A randomized, controlled trial. Ann Surg 2006;244(3): 400–9.

22. Sachdeva AK. Acquiring skills in new procedures and technology: the challenge and the opportunity. Arch Surg 2005;140(4):387–9.
23. Coleman MG, Hanna GB, Kennedy R, et al. The national training programme for laparoscopic colorectal surgery in England: a new training paradigm. Colorectal Dis 2011;13(6):614–6.
24. Miskovic D, Ni M, Wyles SM, et al. Is competency assessment at the specialist level achievable? A study for the national training programme in laparoscopic colorectal surgery in England. Ann Surg 2013;257(3):476–82.
25. Bass BL, Polk HC, Jones RS, et al. Surgical privileging and credentialing: a report of a discussion and study group of the American Surgical Association. J Am Coll Surg 2009;209(3):396–404.
26. The American Board of Surgery. Maintenance of Certification: guidelines on re-entry to surgical practice. Available at: http://www.absurgery.org/default.jsp?policypracticereentry. Accessed September 12, 2015.
27. American Medical Association. Physician re-entry. Available at: http://www.ama-assn.org/ama/pub/education-careers/finding-position/physician-reentry.page?#. Accessed September 12, 2015.
28. Neily J, Mills PD, Young-Xu Y, et al. Association between implementation of a medical team training program and surgical mortality. JAMA 2010;304(15):1693–700.
29. Forse RA, Bramble JD, McQuillan R. Team training can improve operating room performance. Surgery 2011;150(4):771–8.
30. Sachdeva AK, Pellegrini CA, Johnson KA. Support for simulation-based surgical education through American College of Surgeons-Accredited Education Institutes. World J Surg 2008;32(2):196–207.
31. Fann JI, Calhoon JH, Carpenter AJ, et al. Simulation in coronary artery anastomosis early in cardiothoracic surgical residency training: the boot camp experience. J Thorac Cardiovasc Surg 2010;139(5):1275–81.

The Aging Surgeon

Implications for the Workforce, the Surgeon, and the Patient

Paul J. Schenarts, MD*, Samuel Cemaj, MD

KEYWORDS

• Surgeon • Aging • Retirement • Outcomes

KEY POINTS

- The surgical workforce is aging. Nearly one-third of currently active surgeons are older than 55 years.
- Surgeons undergo the same age-related decline in neurocognitive, sensory, and neuromuscular function as the remainder of society; however, this decline may have a negative impact on patient care.
- The complexity of surgical practice and the surgical literature is expanding at an exponential rate. However, the physiologic impairments associated with aging limit the aging surgeon's ability to keep up. As a result, older surgeons frequently have a knowledge deficit and do not fully adhere to modern standards of care.
- Although greater experience might be considered a benefit, an evolving body of literature shows that there is an inverse and paradoxic relationship between greater experience and quality patient outcomes.

According to the US Department of Health and Human Services, the expected lifespan of a baby born in 2010 is 78.7 years, and this life expectancy is anticipated to continue to increase.[1] Not only will the surgeon of the future care for a greater number of elderly patients, the number of elder surgeons will also increase. Surgeons are not immune to the age-related deterioration of neurocognitive, sensory, and motor functions. Likewise, medical and psychiatric conditions common in the elderly also impact aging surgeons. Although greater clinical experience may benefit patients, these age-related physiologic changes may also paradoxically result in poor patient outcomes. Because aging surgeons are reluctant to abandon their career, alterative pathways to contribute need to be considered.[2]

Department of Surgery, University of Nebraska, College of Medicine, 983280 Nebraska Medical Center, Omaha, NE 68198-3280, USA
* Corresponding author.
E-mail address: paul.schenarts@unmc.edu

Surg Clin N Am 96 (2016) 129–138
http://dx.doi.org/10.1016/j.suc.2015.09.009
0039-6109/16/$ – see front matter © 2016 Elsevier Inc. All rights reserved.

THE AGING OF THE SURGICAL WORKFORCE

The surgical workforce is aging. According to the American Medical Association, 18% of practicing physicians are older than 65 years.[3] It is estimated that in the United States, nearly one-third of surgeons currently in practice are older than 55 years.[4] This same trend also being seen in other countries. In Australia, the average age of a surgeon is 52 years with 19% of active surgeons being 65 years or older.[5] Not only are surgeons aging, they are doing so at an exponential rate, with the number of Australian surgeons age 65 years and older increasing by 11% between 2011 and 2012.[6] Complicating matters further, the age at which surgeons retire is also increasing.[7] The larger number of nontraditional medical students, increasing duration of residency training (ie, orthopedic surgery), and the exponential increase in fellowship training means those just entering practice are starting at an age much older than those in previous generations.[8]

The graying of the surgical work force is affecting different patient populations more than others. Using data from the 2009 American Medical Association Physician Masterfile and the American Board of Medical Specialties, Walker and colleagues[4] studied 137,426 surgeons. They found that the specialties of urology and thoracic surgery had the oldest surgeons, with median ages of 52 and 51 years, respectively. Orthopedic, ophthalmic, and plastic surgeons all had a median age of 50 years or older, with 34% to 37% of surgeons older than 55 years. Across all subspecialties, rural surgeons are significantly older compared with their urban counterparts. Geographically, the Midwest has the lowest percentage of surgeons older than 55 years (32%), whereas the West has the highest proportion of older surgeons (35%).[4]

US medical schools have also experienced the impact of aging. In 1967, the average faculty age was 41.7 years; this increased to 44.7 years in 1987 and then 48.5 years in 2007. The percentage of all faculty members older than 55 years was 9% in 1967, 19% in 1987, and 29% in 2007.[9] Between 1967 and 2007, there has been a 7-fold increase in the number of US medical school faculty; however, the starting faculty members are significantly older. As a result, the recruited faculty may not be young enough to offset the overall aging of the retained faculty.[9] The rate of attrition for full professors, who would logically be older, is much slower than that seen for younger assistant and associate professors.[10] Most National Institutes of Health–funded research occurs at medical schools; in parallel with the aging of medical school faculty, the age distribution of National Institutes of Health principal investigators is also increasing. In 1980, less than 1% of principal investigators were older than 65 years but in 2012 that number had increased to 7%.[11]

SURGEONS AND RETIREMENT

The issue of when to transition from practice to retirement is not unique to surgeons. However, the physical and cognitive demands of surgical procedures and perioperative care make the timely retirement of an aging surgeon a public health concern. In the United States, mandated retirement on the grounds of age alone is illegal based on the Age Discrimination in Employment Act of 1967. Additionally, mandatory retirement based on age does not fit well with the universally accepted understanding that onset of cognitive or physical decline is a physiologic process occurring in different individuals at different rates, not a light switch that turns off at a specific age. In contrast, in the commercial airline industry, commercial pilots face mandatory retirement at 60 years of age; similarly, the retirement age of British Surgeons is 65 years from institutional practice and 70 years from private practice.[12]

At age 60 years, most surgeons continue to work, and 17% continue to operate after 70 years of age.[2] The average age of retirement of a general surgeon in 1984 was 60.5 years of age. By 1995, that age had increased to 63 years.[7] In a classic study of members of the American Surgical Association by Greenfield and Proctor, less than 50% of survey respondents reported having any retirement plan, and, among those who did, 75% planned activities in retirement that involved medicine.[2]

There are several potential reasons why surgeons resist retirement. Many surgeons see their own sense of self-value in the ability to perform surgery. In a study of orthopedic surgeons, one-third of respondents reported that the most difficult aspect of retirement was the loss of the role as a surgeon.[13] The all-consuming nature of a surgical practice and the feelings of indispensability, particularly in rural communities, may also be a contributing factor.[14] Other reasons for resistance to retirement include lack of self-esteem, fear of death, resistance to change, loss of financial security, and fear of boredom.[8,15] Further, some doctors feel that their advanced age confers greater credibility, more respect, and better perspective, and nearly one-half feel advanced age gives them greater clinical confidence and competence.[16] An often unrecognized contributing factor for not retiring when the time has arrived may be the inability for the surgeon to perceive his or her own poor performance.

Despite these potential concerns, several studies have documented that most physicians enjoy retirement.[17,18] In a study of 2132 retired surgeons, those who took up postretirement activities outside of medicine were more satisfied than those who remained in medicine in a nonsurgical capacity.[17]

PHYSIOLOGIC CHANGES OF THE AGING SURGEON

Although a surgeon may be the subject of a catastrophic life-changing or life-ending event, the more typical pattern is a slow, insidious deterioration of multiple physiologic processes that impact surgeon performance and ultimately patient care. Further complicating this picture are data documenting that physicians do not adequately look after their own physical health.[19] For example, despite hepatitis B being a major risk of the profession, vaccination rates may be as low as 49%, whereas dentists have nearly a 100% vaccination rate.[20,21]

The attributes of a surgeon could be defined as the ability to think clearly in complex and dynamic situations, while utilizing sensory information to impact patient well-being through the use of dexterity and judgment. Unfortunately, all of these functions decline as a part of the normal aging process.

Decline in Cognition and Neuromuscular Function

As a consequence of normal aging, there is a predictable decline in neurocognitive function across many different domains. Although there are individual variations, of particular concern to the surgeon is the decline in the ability to focus attention, the ability to process and correlate information, and native intelligence.[22] Other examples of age-related deterioration include fluid intelligence (adaptive thinking and clinical reasoning), processing speed, episodic memory (incorporating personally experienced events), and manual dexterity.[23] The aging process also specifically affects cognitive speed and short-term memory and the ability to arrive at a solution for a new type of problem.[24] Reaction time, the time required to move in response to a stimulus, also declines with age, albeit slowly.[8] Although many of these changes are thought to occur at very advanced age, these changes may be seen in older but not yet elderly physicians. In a study of nonsurgeons (psychiatrists) older than 55 years, 10% reported poor memory.[16]

In addition to these physiologic changes, there are also anatomic changes with advancing age. There is a preferential shrinkage of the frontal lobe. Although not well correlated with cognitive decline, the frontal lobes are responsible for the exercise of judgment and insight. Deterioration of these executive functions are particularly relevant in clinical practice.[25]

Further complicating the normal cognitive changes of progressive aging is the development of chronic medical illnesses. Cardiovascular disease, depression, dementia, and excessive alcohol use all further complicate the normal decline in neurocognitive function.[26]

Although these areas of decline are important, there are some neurocognitive functions that are preserved despite aging. Verbal skills and semantic memory (knowledge of facts and meanings) remain intact.[23,27] Crystallized intelligence (the cumulative end product of information acquired over time, hence, clinical wisdom) is also preserved.[24] Additionally, some evidence suggests older physicians may be superior at the use of nonanalytic diagnostic strategies, such as pattern recognition.[28]

Sensory Impairment

Age-related decline in hearing, visual acuity, depth perception, and color discrimination all could negatively impact surgeon performance.[23] With advancing age, there is a progressive hardening and yellowing of the lens of the eye and pupillary shrinkage. The result is that workers older than 55 years require 100% more illumination for optimal performance.[15]

Impact of Prolonged Physical and Psychological Stress

The practice of medicine in general, and surgery in particular, is both physically and mentally challenging. Prolonged, repetitive exposure to these stressors is bound to have consequences. In a study of nonsurgeons older than 55 years, 27% reported that fatigue interfered with their work.[16] The physical nature of surgical work also takes its toll. For example, up to 87% of laparoscopic surgeons reported physical complaints, of which the strongest predictor was high case volume. However, even low case volume surgeons experienced eye and back complaints.[29]

Mental or emotional exhaustion may also take a toll. As one progresses through a career, symptoms of burnout may appear. In addition to feelings of depersonalization and reduced sense of personal accomplishment, a host of other medical conditions, such as anxiety, depression, substance abuse, sleep disturbance, lowered immunity, and possibly ischemic heart disease, may further impair the aging surgeon's performance.[30]

The incidence of burnout in surgeons of all age groups is as high as 40% according to a survey of 8000 members of the American College of Surgeons in 2008. This burnout is associated with suicidal ideation in up to 6.4% (1.5–3 times more than that in the general population).[31]

One of the major contributing factors to burnout is chronic sleep deprivation.[30] Although concerns about patient safety have resulted in duty hour restrictions for trainees, heretofore there has not been any focus on this issue for the aging surgeon, who would be expected to have even less physical reserve and who is not subject to the same oversight as younger trainees.

The question about older surgeons being more at risk for burnout is, however, controversial. Peisah and colleagues[32] found that older practitioners experienced less burnout, and this was attributed to lessons learned over the course of their careers (although women might be more vulnerable to burnout).

Psychiatric Illness

The presence of mental and psychiatric disease has an increased incidence in the elderly physician. In a study of impairment in older doctors, 54% were found to have cognitive impairment or dementia, including 12% with frank dementia; 22% had depression, 17% had a neurodegenerative disease, and 29% had some form of substance abuse (of which, 20% had alcohol abuse and 17% had opiate abuse).[28] Another Australian study of 11,379 practitioners found nearly 10% of surgeons reported having suicidal ideation in the previous year. In the same study 2.5% of surgeons had serious psychological distress, and 20.5% had a high likelihood of a minor psychiatric disorder.[33] This same study reported that physicians had a higher degree of denial with regard to the impact illness was having on their performance.

Neurocognitive Testing

Several tests have been developed that could be used to monitor cognitive function of the aging surgeon. In particular, the MicroCog, which is designed to measure reactivity, attention, numeric recall, verbal memory, visiospatial facility reasoning, and mental calculation, has been suggested as a method to detect impaired competence in surgeons.[12] However, although good scores on items such as visuospatial facility and reaction times would be important for surgeons, there have been no studies correlating good or bad scores with actual clinical outcomes.[8] Another useful test may be the game of chess. Playing chess has several similarities to surgery, such as complexity, time pressure, and rewards or penalties for decisions made. These results can easily be objectified based on wins and losses adjusted for the skill of the opponent. Unfortunately, similar to the MicroCog, there is no evidence that a chess rating correlates with clinical outcomes.[8] The use of the Mini Mental Status Exam has been explored, but there is a ceiling effect, so it may not be useful in detecting impairment among physicians.[28,34]

DIFFICULTY TEACHING "OLD DOGS NEW TRICKS"

Current clinical practice is vastly different than formal educational training obtained by the older surgeon. The remoteness of education or the timeframe between ending formal education and current practice is significant for the aging surgeon. Based on the average older surgeon entering practice at age 31 years, remoteness of education has been estimated to be 31 years minus the surgeon's age.[8] Consider the example of orthopedic surgery. Over the last 25 years, essentially every surgical treatment has changed. Femoral shaft fractures, treated with 6 weeks of traction, followed by another 6 weeks in a plaster cast were first replaced with plate fixation, and that technique has been abandoned for locked intramedullary nailing.[8] Other examples of evolving techniques over the last several decades include laparoscopic surgery, modern bariatric surgery, nonoperative management of blunt organ trauma, and robotic surgery. The evolution of each of these new techniques requires the older surgeon to learn, embrace, and incorporate them into their daily practice.

Unfortunately, typical neuropsychological changes of advanced age make this learning particularly difficult. The following findings on testing significantly impair learning in this age group: decreased auditory memory, decreased learning abilities, motor and mental slowing, difficulty retaining facts, difficulty reading, and tendency to become more concrete in thinking.[28] These factors contribute to a mentality of "my mind is made up don't confuse me with the facts." The manifestation of this learning impairment may have clinical consequences. In a study of 395 plastic surgeons investigating the role of age on practice patterns in the treatment of melanoma, older surgeons ordered more chemical tests such as 5-S-cyteinyl dopa, which is no longer believed to be helpful, whereas younger surgeons ordered chemical tests currently thought to be more useful.[35] In a study of 498 specialized breast surgeons, older surgeons were significantly less likely to perform immediate reconstruction (odds ratio, 5.2) and more likely to feel that immediate breast reconstruction had disadvantages.[36] Despite the multiple advantages of laparoscopy, 2 studies found an inverse relationship between the years in practice, advanced age, and performance of laparoscopy.[37,38] Neumayer and colleagues,[39] however, found that patients of surgeons older than 45 years had increased recurrence rates after laparoscopic hernia repairs. Although the results of these studies suggest concern, it should be noted they were all performed more than a decade ago. However, these studies do document the difficulties with older surgeons learning new surgical techniques.

THE GREAT PARADOX OF THE AGING SURGEON: GREATER EXPERIENCE BUT WORSE CLINICAL PERFORMANCE

Evaluation of quality of performance metrics has become a central focus across all of medical practice. It would be reasonable to assume that older physicians who have greater experience would provide better quality care and have improved outcomes. Evolving data, however, paradoxically finds the opposite to be true. In a comprehensive, carefully constructed systematic review, Choudhry and colleagues[40] found that physicians who have been in practice longer are at risk for providing lower quality care. In their investigation, 12 studies found an inverse relationship between years of experience and knowledge base.[40] An example of interest was a study of surgeons and anesthesiologists assessing knowledge of the indications for and the risks associated with blood transfusion. In that study, Salem-Schatz and colleagues[41] found a highly significant association between knowledge deficit and the number of years in practice. Given this, it is not surprising that older surgeons have an inferior performance on recertification examinations.[42] Choudhry and colleagues[40] also found that most (63%) studies investigating adherence to standards of practice for diagnosis, screening, and prevention found the longer a physician is in practice, the less likely they are to adhere to standards. A large study assessing adherence to nationally established cancer screening guidelines found that physicians who graduated 20 years earlier were less likely to adhere to these recommendations.[43] A similar trend was also seen with adherence to standards of appropriate therapy. A full 74% of studies found a negative association between physician age and adherence to standards of therapeutic care.[40] Not only are older physicians less likely to incorporate new treatment strategies, they are also more likely to prescribe inappropriate medications.[44,45]

Unfortunately, a growing body of literature suggests that more experienced physicians and surgeons paradoxically have worse clinical outcomes.[39,40,46–50] Although Burns and Wholey[51] found no relationship between physician age and mortality, they did find that after adjusting for comorbid conditions, patients of physicians of greater experience did have a longer hospital length of stay. In contrast, another more recent systematic review found that increased volume and greater surgeon experience with specific procedures did result in improved outcome.[52]

ASSURING COMPETENCY AND PHYSICAL AND MENTAL CAPABILITIES
Why Problem Surgeons Are Not Identified

Assuring surgeon competence is the responsibility of 2 agencies. The respective Board, and subspecialty board, of Medicine and Surgery have traditionally been focused on determining suitability for entrance into practice but have recently taken greater responsibility for ongoing monitoring of competence through more robust maintenance of certification requirements.[53] Although state boards provide a mechanism for discipline in the event of a major untoward event, the aging surgeon tends to fail gradually, and this issue may remain undetected. There are conflicting data on whether older physicians are overrepresented among those referred to regulatory agencies.[14] A study of allopathic physicians in Oklahoma found that the proportion of physicians disciplined increased with each successive 10-year interval since first licensure.[54] Individual hospitals may also identify older surgeons at risk for unsafe practice. However, because health care is a redundant system, the errors of an individual may not be obvious. Even if obvious, hospitals, particularly small rural hospitals, may have a potential conflict of interest in disciplining the surgeon because of financial concerns.

Assuring Competent Care

As outlined above, older surgeons may suffer from a knowledge deficit and not adhere to modern standards of care.[40] These concerns could be addressed easily with the recent changes toward a more robust recertification program. Unfortunately, dependence on peer review or self-reporting may not be useful, as there are political difficulties in approaching a senior surgeon, and most senior surgeons are not actually providing care with a surgeon of equal authority or experience.

Evaluating Physical and Mental Capabilities

Older surgeons fail as the result of biology, rather than willful misconduct. The surgeon has no control over the deterioration of cognitive function, reaction time, dexterity, and evolution of medical or psychiatric disease. Currently, there is no required battery of neurocognitive or physical testing of older surgeons to remain in practice. Trunkey and Botney[12] have outlined a schema for such an evaluation. In brief, this schema involves obtaining a complete medical history, physical examination, and electrocardiogram at age 50 years. In addition, some measure of neurocognitive function, such as the MicroCog Test would be performed. This process would be repeated every 2 years until age 60 and annually thereafter. Trunkey and Botney[12] also suggest that a recertification examination be conducted every 3 years after the age of 55 with the emphasis on recent concepts and new knowledge. Others have added the importance of mental health screening to this paradigm.[32]

Katlic and associates[55] propose a 2-day comprehensive multidisciplinary, objective, and confidential evaluation of a surgeon's physical and cognitive function, designed to protect surgeons from an unreliable or arbitrary evaluation and to identify a treatable disorder. This program is also helpful in determining when it is time to retire.

Adaptive Strategies

As surgeons age, their practice patterns change. Bieliauskas and colleagues[56] found that as they age, surgeons reduce the volume and complexity of cases. Older physicians also adapt to the decline in cognitive function by allocating more time to each patient, increasing use of memory aids, working with others, and increasingly seeking second opinions.[14,57] The workplace may also adapt to meet the needs of the aging physician. In 2009, the American College of Emergency Physicians recommended that older physicians work weekend day shifts instead if night shifts, more consistent shifts at a set time of day or night, and fewer consecutive shifts and exchange clinical responsibilities for teaching or administrative duties.[58] Ceasing all night calls and reducing overall duty hours after a specified age, similar to what is now required of interns, may also be an option.

UTILIZING THE AGING SURGEON

As surgeons progress toward the end of their operative career, they continue to need intellectual stimulation and feel the obligation to continue contributing. One potential outlet for the surgeon emeritus is teaching. Given the concerns presented earlier about knowledge deficits and nonstandard practices of aging surgeons, the assignment of educational roles needs to be considered carefully. Whereas clinical teaching of residents may not be appropriate, teaching anatomy, history, and physical examination skills and basic surgical skills could be of great benefit to surgeons and students alike.[59]

Sir William Osler once said: "The teacher's life should have three periods, study until age twenty-five, investigation until forty, profession until sixty, at which age I would have him retired on a double allowance."[60]

REFERENCES

1. Arias E. United states life tables, 2010. Natl Vital Stat Rep 2014;63(7):1–63.
2. Greenfield LJ, Proctor MC. Attitudes towards retirement. A survey of the American Surgical Association. Ann Surg 1994;220(3):382–90.
3. Smart DR. Physician characteristics and distribution in the US-2006. Chicago: American Medical Association; 2006.
4. Walker E, Poley S, Ricketts T. The aging surgeon population, vol. 5. Chapel Hill (NC): American College of Surgeons Research Institute; 2010.
5. Australian Institute of Health & Welfare. Medical workforce 2012. Canberra (Australia): AIW; 2014. National Health Workforce Series no.8. Cat. No. HWL 54.
6. Royal Australasian College of Surgeons. Surgical workforce projection to 2025 (for Australia). 2012.
7. Jonasson O, Kwakwa F. Retirement age and the work force in general surgery. Ann Surg 1996;224:574–82.
8. Blasier RB. The problem of the aging surgeon. When surgeon age becomes a surgical risk factor. Clin Orthop Relat Res 2009;467:402–11.
9. Alexander H, Liu CQ. 4th edition. The aging of full-time U.S. medical school faculty: 1967-2007, vol. 9. Washington, DC: Association of American Medical Colleges; 2009.
10. Liu CQ, Morrison E. 2nd edition. U.S. medical school full-time faculty attrition, vol. 14. Washington, DC: Association of American Medical Colleges; 2014.
11. Rocky S. Age distribution of princireport and medical school faculty. 2012. Available at: http://nexus.od.nih.giv/all/2012/02/13age-distribution-of-nih-prinipal-investigators-and-medical-school-faculty. Accessed May 9, 2015.
12. Trunkey DD, Botney R. Assessing competency: A tale of two professions. J Am Coll Surg 2001;192:385–95.
13. Ritter MA, Austrom MG, Zhou H, et al. Retirement from orthopaedic surgery. J Bone Joint Surg Am 1999;81:414–8.
14. Adler RG, Constaninou C. Knowing-or not knowing-when to stop: cognitive decline in ageing doctors. Med J Aust 2008;189:622–4.
15. Rovit RL. To everything there is a season and a time to every purpose: retirement and the neurosurgeon. J Neurosurg 2004;100:1123–9.
16. Draper B, Winfield S, Luscombe G. The older psychiatrist and retirement. Int J Geriatr Psychiatry 1997;12:233–9.

17. Miscall BG, Tompkins RK, Greenfield LJ. ACS survey explores retirement and the surgeon. Bull Am Coll Surg 1996;81:18–25.
18. Virshup B, Coombs RH. Physicians' adjustment to retirement. West J Med 1993; 158:142–4.
19. Kay MP, Mitchell GK, De Mar CB. Doctors do not adequately look after their own physical health. MJA 2004;181:368–70.
20. Department of Health and Ageing. Australian immunization handbook. 8th edition. Canberra (Australia): National Health and Medical Research Council; 2003.
21. Couts T, Cannata S, Nira M, et al. Hepatitis B vaccine. Med J Aust 1992;156:294 [letter].
22. Greenfield LJ, Proctor MC. When should a surgeon retire? Adv Surg 1999;32: 385–93.
23. Peisah C, Willheml K. The impaired aging doctor. Intern Med J 2002;32:457–9.
24. Catte RB. Theory of fluid and crystalized intelligence: a critical experiment. J Educ Psychol 1963;54:1–22.
25. Trollor JN, Valenzula MJ. Brain ageing in the new millennium. Aust N Z J Psychiatry 2001;35:788–805.
26. Skowronski GA, Perisah C. The greying intensivist: ageing and medical practice-everyone's problem. MJA 2012;196:505–7.
27. Turnbull J, Cunnington J, Unsal A, et al. Competence and cognitive difficulty in physicians: a follow up study. Acad Med 2006;81:915–91.
28. Peisah C, Willhelm K. Physician don't heal thyself: a descriptive study of impaired older doctors. Int Psychogeriatr 2007;19:974–84.
29. Park A, Lee G, Seagull J, et al. Patients benefit while surgeons suffer: an impending epidemic. J Am Coll Surg 2010;210:306–13.
30. Jarral OA, Baig K, Shetty K, et al. Sleep deprivation leads to burnout and cardiothoracic surgeons have to deal with its consequences. Int J Cardiol 2015;179:70–2.
31. Shanafelt TD, Balch CM, Bechamps GJ, et al. Burnout and career among American surgeons. Ann Surg 2009;250:463–71.
32. Peisah C, Wijeratne C, Waxman B, et al. Adaptive ageing surgeons. ANZ J Surg 2014;84:311–5.
33. Beyond blue. National mental health survey of doctors and medical students. Available at: https://www.beyondblue.org.au/docs/default-source/research-project-files/bl1132-report–nmhdmss-full-report_web.pdf?sfvrsn=2. Accessed January 30, 2014.
34. Ihl R, Frolich L, Dierks T, et al. Differential validity of psychometric tests in dementia of the Alzheimer type. Psychiatry Rev 1992;44:93–106.
35. Margenthaler JA, Johnson DY, Virgo KS, et al. Evaluation of patients with clinically suspected melanoma recurrence: current practice patterns of plastic surgeons. Int J Oncol 2002;21:591–6.
36. Callaghan CJ, Couto E, Kerin MJ, et al. Breast reconstruction in the United Kingdom and Ireland. Br J Surg 2002;89:335–40.
37. Wang DS, Winfield HN. Survey of urological laproscopic practice patterns in the widwest. J Urol 2004;172:2282–6.
38. Ahmad S, Lettsome L, Schurit A. The role of laparoscopy in the management of groin hernia. JSLS 1998;2:169–73.
39. Neumayer LA, Gawnda AA, Wang J, Giobbie-Hurder A, et al. Proficiency of surgeons in inguinal hernia repair: effect of experience and age. Ann Surg 2005;242:344–8.
40. Choudhry NK, Fletcher RH, Soumerai SB. Systematic review: the relationship between clinical experience and quality of health care. Ann Intern Med 2005;142: 260–73.

41. Salem-Schatz SR, Avorn J, Soumerai SB. Influence of clinical knowledge, organizational context and practice style on transfusion decision making. Implications for practice change strategies. JAMA 1990;264:476–83.
42. Cruft GE, Humphreys JW Jr, Hermann RE, et al. Recertification in surgery, 1980. Arch Surg 1981;16:1093–6.
43. Czaja R, McFall SL, Warnecke RB, et al. Preferences of community physicians for cancer screening guidelines. Ann Intern Med 1994;120:602–8.
44. Stolley PD, Becker MH, Lasagna L, et al. The relationship between physician characteristics and prescribing appropriateness. Med Care 1972;10:17–8.
45. Rhee SO. Factors determining the quality of physician performance in patient care. Med Care 1976;14:733–50.
46. Waljee JF, Greenfield LJ, Dimick JB, et al. Surgeon age and operative mortality in the United States. Ann Surg 2006;224:353–62.
47. O'Neill L, Lanska DJ, Hartz A. Surgeon cahracteristics associated with mortality and morbidity following carotid endarterectomy. Neurolog 2000;55:773–81.
48. Hartz AJ, Kuhn EM, Pulido J. Prestige of training programs and experience of bypass surgeons as factors in adjusted mortality rates. Med Care 1999;37:93–103.
49. Heck DA, Robinson RL, Partridge CM, et al. Patient outcomes after knee replacement. Clin Orthop Relat Res 1998;356:93–110.
50. Duclos A, Peix JL, Colin C, et al. Influence of experience on performance of individual surgeons in thyroid surgery: prospective cross sectional multicenter study. BMJ 2012;344:1–11.
51. Burns LR, Wholey DR. The effects of patient, hospital and physician characteristics on length of stay and mortality. Med Care 1991;29:251–71.
52. Maruthappu M, Gilbert BJ, El-Haarasis MA, et al. The influence of volume and experience on individual performance: a systematic review. Ann Surg 2015;261:642–7.
53. Callender GG, Kaplan BJ, White RL, et al. Maintenance of certification: what everyone needs to know. Ann Surg Oncol 2015;22:1051–4.
54. Khaliq AA, Dimassi H, Huang CY, et al. Disciplinary action against physicians: who is likely to get disciplined? Am J Med 2005;118:773–7.
55. Katlic MR, Coleman J. The aging surgeon. Ann Surg 2014;260:199–201.
56. Bieliauskas LA, Langenecker S, Graver C, et al. Cognitive changes and retirement among senior surgeons (CRASS): results from the CCRASS study. J Am Coll Surg 2008;207:69–79.
57. Peisah C, Gautam M, Goldstein MZ. Medical masters: a pilot stud of adaptive ageing in physicians. Aust J Ageing 2009;28:134–8.
58. American College of Emergency Physicians. Considerations for emergency physicians in pre-retirement years. Ann Emerg Med 2009;5:641.
59. Kirk RM. The retired surgeon: a potential teaching resource. Ann R Coll Surg Engl 1997;79(suppl):73–4.
60. Bliss M. William Osler: a life in medicine. New York: Oxford University Press; 1999.

Forks in the Road

The Assessment of Surgeons from the American Board of Surgery Perspective

Jo Buyske, MD[a,b]

KEYWORDS

- Assessment • Certification • Maintenance of certification • Diplomate
- Surgical resident • Re-entry • Boot camp

KEY POINTS

- The American Board of Surgery (ABS) serves both the public and the profession.
- Certification is the culmination of multiple assessments beginning during residency. Some assessments can be embedded in residency as part of a continuum of learning and assessment.
- Continued learning and assessment after formal training is completed are critical to ensure the quality of the profession and to enhance the public trust.

The ABS exists to protect the public and enhance the profession. The original ABS Booklet of Information from 1937 includes the following explanation: "This (the formation of the ABS) is to be done for the protection of the public and the good of the specialty." The ABS works to fulfill this charge by assessing surgeons with the best tools available. Assessment of surgeons, similar to the field of surgery itself, is something that changes over time…New tools, new techniques, and new understanding emerge.

There are 4 distinct periods of learning during the career of a surgeon. The first period is in medical school, during the core surgery clerkship and during the fourth year. Ideally, during this period, basic knowledge and some early skills and judgment are acquired so that the first-day resident is prepared to suture a wound, tie a knot, place a bladder catheter, or answer a call about a postoperative patient. Historically, the ABS has had no role in the medical school portion of surgical training.

The second period is during surgical residency. Until recently, the role of the ABS during residency has been limited. In conjunction with the Residency Review Committee for Surgery (RRC-S) of the Accreditation Council for Graduate Medical Education (ACGME), the ABS sets training standards for surgical residency. The ACGME

Disclosure: Full-time salaried employee of the American Board of Surgery.
[a] American Board of Surgery, 1617 John F. Kennedy Boulevard, Suite 860, Philadelphia, PA 19103, USA; [b] University of Pennsylvania School of Medicine, 3400 Spruce Street, Philadelphia, PA 19104, USA
E-mail address: jbuyske@absurgery.org

Surg Clin N Am 96 (2016) 139–146
http://dx.doi.org/10.1016/j.suc.2015.09.010
0039-6109/16/$ – see front matter
surgical.theclinics.com

accredits programs that adhere to these standards; the ABS certifies individuals who successfully complete these programs and successfully pass the Qualifying Examination and Certifying Examination of the ABS. Ideally, during residency trainees acquire the skills necessary to practice independently or to pursue further training in a specialty.

The third period, which most but not all surgeons undertake, is postresidency (or, in the case of surgical critical care, during residency) fellowship. During fellowship training, a particular skill or knowledge set is honed. Some fellowships culminate in ABS or other American Board of Medical Specialties (ABMS) assessment and, if successful, certification. Others function outside of the ACGME/ABS axis and serve as additional training under other independent organizations. Ideally, fellowship training allows for mastery of a subspecialty of general surgery.

The fourth period is the longest and is the period from the end of formal training until retirement. During this period, both knowledge and skills continue to develop. Ideally the practicing surgeon also keeps abreast of changing information and technology and adapts their practice to accommodate new information. The role of the ABS during this phase of a surgical lifetime has evolved from nothing prior to 1976 to Maintenance of Certification (MOC) beginning in 2005.

HISTORY

Initially, the ABS focused exclusively on one point in time: the moment when a surgeon had completed training and was poised to begin practice. The first period of learning, medical school, was left to medical schools, with no oversight or interaction with the boards. The years of residency, likewise, were spent out of sight of the ABS, other than that they occurred in programs where the standards had been developed with the ABS as a lead in defining those standards.

The ABS interaction with surgeons began at the end of residency, when an applicant makes contact with the board for the first time by applying for formal assessment, ideally culminating in certification. The assessment consisted of 3 parts: an application testifying to the details and experience acquired in training; part I, a written or qualifying examination; and part II, an oral or certifying examination. Originally there was also a practical component of Part II, consisting of an observed operation and witnessed patient examinations, among other things, but the use of live patients was discontinued in the 1950s. Certification was for life: once the process demonstrated adequate training (application), knowledge (the written examination), and judgment (the oral examination), a surgeon was certified. Those who were certified were free to practice and to carry that certificate for life.

TIME-LIMITED CERTIFICATES AND RECERTIFICATION

More recently, the ABS has concerned itself with the continuum of training across the lifetime of a surgeon. The first step toward this was the institution of time-limited certificates. As early as 1940, the Commission on Graduate Medical Education made the argument that the explosive growth in medical knowledge made point-in-time, lifetime certification insufficient to assure current knowledge and practice. The American Board of Family Practice (later the American Board of Family Medicine) was the first to adopt time-limited certification, in 1970. The ABS quickly followed suit, becoming the second board to require time-limited certificates, in 1976 (with an initial foray into that arena with time-limited certificates in pediatric surgery in 1973).

Subsequent experience with requirements for recertification have validated the need for time-limited certificates. It quickly became apparent, as suspected, that a surgeon's knowledge base changes over the years and that a surgeon who has been out of training for 10, 20, or 30 years is not the same as a fresh trainee. This is demonstrated by the variation seen in the scores and failure rate on the Recertification Examination (now MOC) of the ABS. Surgeons who are 10 years away from their initial certification fail the examination at a rate of 3.4%. Those who are 20 years out fail at 7.9%, and those 30 years out fail at 10.9%. Just recently, there have been some 40 year cohort examinees, who failed at a rate of 22% (**Table 1**). This has served to reinforce the tenet that more frequent assessment of knowledge is necessary and appropriate to fulfill the dual charges of protecting the public and enhancing the profession. There may be several factors in the increasing failure rate over time. Narrowed field of practice may lead to loss of familiarity with some areas of surgery. Dual certification such that the specialty certification has more importance to the surgeon may make studying for the surgery examination less pressing. Nevertheless, the variation in scores supports the idea that a surgeon 10 years out of residency is not the same as a surgeon 30 or 40 years out of residency, and it is incumbent on the ABS to recognize that fact in its assessment and certification procedures.

Time-limited certificates and recertification were the first steps in the ABS addressing the full lifetime of learning in the practice of surgeons.

Table 1
American Board of Surgery diplomate cohort fail rates on the recertification examination or maintenance of certification examination in surgery, 1995–2014

	10 Years		20 Years		30 Years		Total	
	N	Fail (%)	N	Fail (%)	N	Fail (%)	N	Fail (%)
1995	857	3.6	252	8.7	—	—	1109	4.8
1996	872	4.5	395	6.8	—	—	1267	5.2
1997	830	2.5	584	7.7	—	—	1414	4.7
1998	796	3.0	678	9.4	—	—	1474	6.0
1999	846	3.2	773	10.5	—	—	1619	6.7
2000	639	3.3	584	12.5	—	—	1223	7.7
2001	728	2.6	642	11.7	—	—	1370	6.9
2002	759	4.3	596	11.9	—	—	1355	7.7
2003	816	3.9	650	16.2	23	43.5	1489	9.9
2004	800	3.8	665	9.9	98	22.4	1563	7.5
2005	784	4.5	611	9.3	160	18.8	1555	7.8
2006	753	4.5	633	6.2	192	9.4	1578	5.8
2007	764	3.4	665	6.2	275	12.7	1703	6.0
2008	768	3.1	642	6.4	340	11.2	1750	5.9
2009	868	4.0	729	4.1	470	11.1	2067	5.7
2010	898	2.6	678	4.0	451	11.1	2027	4.9
2011	842	2.5	627	4.8	426	9.2	1895	4.7
2012	782	1.9	619	2.9	404	7.4	1826	3.7
2013	872	2.8	680	4.6	364	9.1	1932	4.8
2014	604	3.1	520	3.7	315	8.3	1462	4.7
TOTAL	15,878	3.4	12,225	7.9	3518	10.9	31,681[a]	6.0

[a] 2012 to 2014 = 59 candidates, 40-year cohort, 22.0% fail.

MAINTENANCE OF CERTIFICATION

The ABMS is a federation of 24 member boards who have voluntarily agreed to cooperate around standards and best practices in certification. The focus of the ABMS is in improving the quality of health care by supporting the lifelong professional development of physicians. The member boards of the ABMS are listed in **Table 2**.

In 2005 all member boards of the ABMS launched MOC to improve on the standards set by a 10-year cycle of episodic recertification. Each board developed the details of its own program, according to overarching standards set by the ABMS. The ABS was an early leader in MOC.

The ABS MOC program incorporates much of what was already being done with recertification. MOC is divided into 4 parts. Part 1 addresses professionalism, and, as with recertification, the ABS requires evidence of an unrestricted state license to practice medicine, hospital credentials, and testimonials from the chair of surgery and chair of the credentials committee. Part 2 addresses lifelong learning, and, as with recertification, there is a requirement for continuing medical education (CME) credits. ABS MOC requires self-assessment CME, which sets a higher bar for accountability than the more passive learning of traditional CME required for recertification. Part 3, a secure assessment of medical knowledge, remains unchanged. Under MOC, the Recertification Examination of the ABS becomes the MOC Examination

Table 2 American Board of Medical Specialties member boards and year in which they were approved	
Board	**Year**
American Board of Ophthalmology	1917
American Board of Otolaryngology	1924
American Board of Obstetrics and Gynecology	1930
American Board of Dermatology	1932
American Board of Orthopaedic Surgery	1935
American Board of Pediatrics	1935
American Board of Psychiatry and Neurology	1935
American Board of Radiology	1935
American Board of Urology	1935
American Board of Internal Medicine	1936
American Board of Pathology	1936
American Board of Surgery	1937
American Board of Neurologic Surgery	1940
American Board of Anesthesiology	1941
American Board of Plastic Surgery	1941
American Board of Physical Medicine and Rehabilitation	1947
American Board of Colon and Rectal Surgery	1949
American Board of Preventive Medicine	1949
American Board of Family Practice	1969
American Board of Thoracic Surgery	1970
American Board of Nuclear Medicine	1971
American Board of Allergy and Immunology	1971
American Board of Emergency Medicine	1979
American Board of Medical Genetics	1991

but remains a secure, multiple-choice, computer-based examination given at 10-year intervals. To be admitted to the MOC Examination, diplomates of the ABS must be in compliance with MOC.

Part 4 of MOC focuses on assessment and improvement of performance in practice. This is not addressed in initial certification nor was it addressed with recertification. It is a laudable target. The ABS recognizes that assessing performance in practice is a complicated undertaking. This is an area of active investigation. As of now, the ABS accepts participation in an outcomes registry as fulfillment of MOC part 4. The best known of such registries is the National Surgical Quality Improvement Program. Other valuable registries from a variety of surgical societies and hospital or government resources are also accepted.

A summary of ABS MOC standards is in **Table 3**.

PREPARATION FOR RESIDENCY

Changes in the culture of medical school training have changed the experience of medical students. Students have essentially no autonomy during medical school, instead being relegated to the position of bystanders and observers. Hours of clinical exposure have become shorter. Surgical clerkships are shorter, anatomy classes have been cut, and hours on call are the exception rather than the rule. As a result, residents arrive at their training institution with less experience and exposure to patient care. The first months of training are thus spent in remediation, which slows the process of learning surgery. Some individual medical schools have independently developed specific rotations, or boot camps, to better prepare medical

Table 3	
American Board of Surgery maintenance of certification program requirements	
Every 3 years, diplomates submit information via the ABS Web site regarding	
Professional standing	Full and unrestricted medical license; hospital or surgical center privileges; contact information for chief of surgery and chair of credentialing where most work in performed
CME activities	90 Hours of Category 1 CME relevant to the practice is required over a 3-year cycle, with at least 60 of the 90 including self-assessment (written or electronic question-and-answer exercise).
	A score of 75% or higher must be required on the self-assessment activity; however, no minimum number of questions is required and repeated attempts are allowed.
	In addition, the ABS waives 60 hours of CME with self-assessment for passing a certifying or MOC Examination given by the ABS or another ABMS board.
Practice assessment participation	Participation in a local, regional, or national outcomes registry or quality assessment program—surgeons are asked to describe how they are meeting this requirement; no data are collected.
Every 10 years, diplomates are required to successfully complete	
MOC Examination in the specialty	Surgeons are eligible to apply for an MOC Examination starting 3 years before their certificate's expiration. A full examination application is required, including a 12-month operative log (case numbers only), reference forms, and CME documentation. Diplomates must be in compliance with MOC to apply.
	For surgeons who hold multiple ABS certificates, this is the only requirement that must be repeated for each certificate.

students for surgical residencies. Participants in those programs have been shown to be more confident and to outperform their nonparticipating peers in the first several months of residency.[1] In response to this situation, several of the leadership groups in surgery, including the ABS, the American College of Surgeons (ACS), the Association of Program Directors in Surgery, and the Association for Surgical Education, produced the "Statement on Surgical Pre-Residency Preparatory Courses."[2] This calls out the need for programs that ensure that all medical students going into surgery have the fundamental skills required for safe and effective patient care on entering residency. These programs should include interactive sessions, simulation sessions teaching basic procedural skills, communication skills, and learner feedback.

SURGICAL RESIDENCY

The leadership of American surgery has been aware for many years that changing times require ongoing vigilance and attention to the standards of residency training. A blue ribbon committee was convened in 2004 to take a focused look at these issues and in 2005 published an article in the *Annals of Surgery*,[3] in which a series of recommendations regarding training and practice in surgery were made. The recommendations of the Flexner Report, widely credited with substantially improving and standardizing medical education in the United States more than 100 years ago, took 10 years to be fully enacted; based on that experience, the process of re-evaluating and improving surgical training is just about on the same timeline for success.

The ABS, too, in conjunction with the ACS, the RRC-S, and the American Surgical Association, has continually looked for ways to improve resident training. This raises the question: are all residencies the same? To measure progress it is essential to have a common baseline. With that in mind, starting in 2010, the ABS engaged in residency in a more active way, inserting requirements for admissibility to the Qualifying Examination into surgical training. This had the goal and effect of making the experience of residencies in different locations more similar, so that improvement could be measured as apples to apples not oranges to apples. The initial set of new requirements included successful completion of Advanced Trauma Life Support, Advanced Cardiovascular Life Support, and Fundamentals of Endoscopic Surgery. These requirements assured that a certain standard of knowledge in these 3 areas—trauma, cardiovascular resuscitation, and laparoscopy—had been met by all residents in the country.

Over the next few years, additional requirements were implemented, including requirements for observed operations and clinical interactions (surprisingly, this had never been formalized as part of residency training); an increase in the number of teaching assistant (TA) cases required (TA cases are those in which a resident takes a more junior resident through a case); a requirement for 250 cases to be done during the first 2 years; and a requirement to complete a curriculum in endoscopic surgery (Fundamentals of Endoscopy Curriculum), culminating in a skills and knowledge test (Fundamentals of Endoscopic Surgery).

The ABS In-Training Examination (ABSITE), has been a long-standing assessment tool provided to the program directors by the ABS. The purpose of the ABSITE is to allow programs to assess their teaching programs compared with other programs and to assess the knowledge level of individual residents. It is not a pass-fail examination but rather is reported by percentile rank as related to other surgical residents in the country in the same year of training. It is intended as a formative assessment tool, not a summative examination. The high quality and value of this examination have been recognized internationally, and as many as 17 other countries in a given year offer the examination to their trainees for similar purposes.

These requirements and assessments, and the role of the ABS in establishing standards in training, are serving to improve the consistency of training across the country. Having established a stable baseline of training makes improvement and measuring of improvement more attainable.

RE-ENTRY TO CLINICAL PRACTICE

Surgeons leave the practice of surgery for a wide variety of reasons. Some suffer from a medical illness or injury, with forced leave from practice as a consequence. Some make a career change, deciding to pursue further education or other interests or passions. Some make the decision to leave for personal reasons, such as caring for a family member, whether a parent, spouse, sibling, or child. In some cases, the surgeon in question has practiced for many years. In other situations, a surgeon may leave after just a year or 2. Not surprisingly, when the illness resolves or stabilizes, or the family situation changes or perhaps the career change does not work out, these surgeons may want to return to the practice of surgery.

Until recently there was no standard pathway for assessing the skills and knowledge of these surgeons, such that they could be safely returned to the practice of surgery. Recognizing this gap, the ABS convened a retreat on the subject and in 2012 published guidelines on re-entry to surgical practice.[4] Each re-entry pathway is individualized, because no 2 situations are the same. The main elements of re-entry include assessment of status of practice at departure; a re-entry pathway constructed by a local champion and addressing all arenas of competency; a proctoring plan; outcomes assessment; and MOC. Individuals work and their champions work with the ABS to develop an appropriate program, taking into account previous years of experience, the nature of the practice prior to leaving surgery, the time elapsed since leaving surgery, and goals for future practice. Re-entry is recommended for surgeons who have been away from clinical practice for 2 or more years. This multilevel assessment is an improvement that has been helpful to both the credentialing bodies of hospitals and the surgeons who seek re-entry.

SUMMARY

Assessment of surgeons at various points in their training is the main charge of the ABS. Although many surgeons equate assessment only with the Qualifying Examination, Certifying Examination, and MOC Examination, assessment is woven throughout the lifetime of surgical practice. Surgeons engage in self-assessment at morbidity and mortality conferences, through personal reflection, and via the self-assessment requirements of MOC. External assessment is provided by teachers and mentors during medical school, residency, practice, and re-entry. Formal assessment in the form of programs, such as Fundamentals of Laparoscopic Surgery, Advanced Trauma Life Support, Advanced Cardiovascular Life Support, Fundamentals of Endoscopic Surgery, operative evaluations, ABSITE, Qualifying Examination, Certifying Examination, and MOC Examination, are only pieces of the whole.

REFERENCES

1. Antonoff MB, Swanson JA, Green CA, et al. The significant impact of a competency-based preparatory course for senior medical students entering surgical residency. Acad Med 2012;87(3):308–19.

2. American Board of Surgery, American College of Surgeons, Association of Program Directors in Surgery, et al. Statement on surgical pre-residency preparatory courses. JAMA Surg 2014;149(11):1198–9.
3. Debas HT, Bass BL, Brennan MF, et al. American Surgical Association blue ribbon committee report on surgical education: 2004. Ann Surg 2005;241(1):1–8.
4. Re-Entry to Surgical Practice. American Board of Surgery website.

Residency Surgical Training at an Independent Academic Medical Center

Jeremiah Jones, MD[a], Richard A. Sidwell, MD[a,b],*

KEYWORDS

- Independent academic medical center • Surgical education • Surgical residency

KEY POINTS

- Surgical residency training at an independent academic medical center has unique advantages and challenges when compared to university and military programs.
- Independent programs are characterized by strong relationships among residents and faculty; this fosters a supportive learning environment.
- Residents at independent programs tend to have earlier operative experience and have more confidence in their skills at the time of graduation.
- Challenges at independent surgery programs include being able to provide the entire spectrum of clinical experiences, maintaining engagement of the teaching faculty, and meeting budgetary requirement.
- With the workforce need for general surgeons, independent training programs will continue to play an integral role.

INTRODUCTION

There are more than 250 general surgery residency training programs in the United States that are accredited by the Accreditation Council for Graduate Medical Education (ACGME). They can be described broadly as 3 different types of programs. Just over half of these training programs are university programs; these are programs where the primary teaching hospital is also a primary teaching site for a medical school. There are a few military training programs that are operated by the United States Armed Forces. The remainder, nearly one-half of the programs, are either not

The authors have nothing to disclose.
[a] Department of Surgical Education, Iowa Methodist Medical Center, 1415 Woodland Avenue, Suite 140, Des Moines, IA 50309, USA; [b] Department of Surgery, University of Iowa Carver College of Medicine, 1500 John Colloton Pavilion, 200 Hawkins Drive, Iowa City, IA 52242, USA
* Corresponding author. Department of Surgical Education, 1415 Woodland Avenue, Suite 140, Des Moines, IA 50309.
E-mail address: rsidwell@iowaclinic.com

Surg Clin N Am 96 (2016) 147–153
http://dx.doi.org/10.1016/j.suc.2015.09.011
0039-6109/16/$ – see front matter © 2016 Elsevier Inc. All rights reserved.
surgical.theclinics.com

affiliated with or are geographically distinct from a university or the military. Although these programs are commonly called *community* programs, it is most proper for them to be referred to as *independent academic medical centers*. This article seeks to explore the benefits and challenges of surgical training at an independent academic medical center. There is a paucity of scientific data objectively comparing training environments. Much of what is known is subjective and experiential in nature.

HISTORY

Community-based surgical education began to arise in the mid-1800s as university physicians grew their surgical practice. When the number of elective operations these physicians were performing increased, some chose to operate at private hospitals rather than a university center. This model became more common. With time more surgeons were recruited to the community environment. Medical students with an interest in a surgical career followed, and the model of community-based surgical education was developed.[1]

ADVANTAGES

Surgical residency training is a long and difficult journey regardless of the type of residency program. Independent programs are typically smaller than university programs in terms of both resident complement and faculty size. This fosters strong relationships among residents and between residents and faculty members, perhaps the most unique aspect of the training environment at independent programs. It is difficult to describe or quantify the esprit de corps of the residency environment, but it is an essential component of a successful program.

In a cross-sectional national survey of surgical residents, Sullivan and colleagues[2] found that residents training at community programs felt better supported by their programs than did residents at university or military programs. This support was seen in both the educational and the personal aspects of the training years. Additionally, the survey found that residents at community programs were less likely to feel that their working environment was causing a strain on family life.

A supportive learning environment where there is a culture of respect among residents and between residents and faculty is of paramount importance for the overall success of a residency program and the residents who train in the program. At the authors' institution, this type of positive environment was found to encourage the residents to achieve. The strong relationship between residents and faculty results in the faculty personally engaged in the success of the residents. In turn, this establishes a set of expectations that the residents are eager to meet. The cycle becomes self-perpetuating, but it is contingent on the culture of respect and the supportive learning environment.

Sullivan and colleagues[2] found that residents at community programs were more likely to report that the program had support structures in place to help them during periods of struggle. Personal and professional challenges are commonplace during the residency years. Understanding the positive learning environment, it is not surprising that independent programs have a lower rate of resident attrition compared with university programs.[3]

Independent programs are characterized by early and broad operative experience with an emphasis on progressive responsibility. At the authors' institution, junior residents are expected to be in the operating room from the start of their intern year. This is combined with, as a general rule, a lack of competition from subspecialty fellows at independent programs. The result is that the resident has early development of technical skills, both open and laparoscopic, which creates operative confidence for the graduating resident. This is supported in the survey by Sullivan and colleagues,[2] where residents at community programs were more satisfied with their operative experience and less likely to have doubts about their operative ability at the time of graduation.

In summary, independent programs have a supporting learning environment with an emphasis on early operative experience. This leads to high resident satisfaction, low attrition, and improved operative confidence at the time of graduation.

CHALLENGES

In 1984 there were 311 general surgery residency programs. By 2004, as noted by Mahmoud and colleagues,[4] this number was reduced to 253 programs. Independent programs disproportionately accounted for the loss of surgical programs. This is largely attributed to the difficulty that some independent programs had meeting the increasing accreditation requirements from the ACGME. This is one example of the challenges faced by independent programs.

It can be difficult for independent academic medical centers to be able to provide the entire spectrum of necessary clinical experiences at their home institution. Experiences in burn surgery, transplant surgery, pediatric surgery, and trauma surgery are common examples of this. Many community programs have agreements with university programs to allow their residents to do specialty rotations at the university that are not possible in home location. Mahmoud and colleagues[4] described this situation, including the lessons learned, where the surgical residents at San Joaquin General Hospital travel approximately 60 miles to the University of California, Davis, to fulfill their transplant and pediatric surgery requirements. This allows the community program to meet an educational gap that would otherwise threaten accreditation. The university program benefits from the increased workforce and a reciprocal experience for their residents at the community hospital. This type of relationship creates stress, however, for the residents from the community program through being away from home for the rotation and having to work in an unfamiliar environment.

Engagement of teaching faculty can be challenging at independent academic medical centers. As a general rule, the faculty members at community programs participate in resident education on a volunteer basis.[5] Clinical instruction (operating room and hospital patients) is usually very good. At times, however, demands for clinical productivity of the private practice surgeon are at odds with resident education. Teaching residents prolongs operative time. Educational conferences, meetings, and skills laboratories compete with clinic and operating room schedules. Pursuit of scholarly activity can be difficult in a community practice. None of these activities generates relative value units, creating a potential financial disadvantage for teaching residents. Community programs constantly seek incentives to encourage faculty participation. Frequently, however, the program relies on intrinsic motivation from individual faculty surgeons.

A complete discussion of institutional cost of a surgical residency program at an independent academic medical center is beyond the scope of this article. There are the traditional costs, including resident salaries and benefits, administrative personnel, and educational facilities. Skills laboratories and simulation centers are now required, which can be particularly challenging in an independent environment. There are many new expenses for programs: Surgical Council on Resident Education curriculum (SCORE), Advanced Trauma Life Support, Fundamentals of Surgery Curriculum, Fundamentals of Laparoscopic Surgery, and Fundamentals of Endoscopic Surgery. These mandates create budgetary challenges for programs. It is critical that the leadership in hospital administration is supportive of the residency program. When compared with physician extenders (nurse practitioners or physician assistants), surgical residents are practical and economical.[6] Although it is difficult to show this on a balance sheet, a surgical residency program at a community hospital improves the quality of patient care.[7]

RESIDENT RECRUITMENT

Perhaps the most crucial task for program directors is to attract and recruit medical students who will be successful surgical residents. This is a particular challenge at independent academic medical centers because they are not primary teaching sites for medical schools and most medical students do not rotate at community hospitals. This means that many students have not had exposure to independent programs when they are beginning the residency application process.

Jarman and colleagues[8] surveyed applicants who were selected to interview at independent programs to determine the resources they used to learn about residency programs. One-third of the respondents reported that they received an imbalanced representation of program types and this bias was nearly uniformly in favor of university programs. Examples of this bias included a narrow scope of university mentors (compared with broadly trained general surgeons), fellowship options, prestige/reputation, and academic and research opportunities. This is not surprising because medical students inherently interact more with surgeons in the university environment; overcoming this bias is a significant challenge for independent programs. This survey also found that applicants rely heavily on individual program Web sites to gather information about independent programs, whereas there is little use of "The Little Red Book,"[9] previously an important resource. Thus, it is critical that program directors ensure that their program's Web site contains current information. On-line conduits for residency information, including the Association for Program Directors in Surgery and Fellowship and Residency Electronic Interactive Database, need to be checked for accuracy.

Independent programs work to increase their exposure to medical students in a variety of ways. Some programs have established clerkship rotations for third-year and/or fourth-year medical students. This allows students to obtain first-hand experience in a different learning environment. Educationally, this approach has been validated. A report from Tufts University School of Medicine showed that some community surgery rotations prepared students better for the shelf examination than did the university hospital. In addition, students thought the quality of their rotations at 2 of the 3 available community hospitals was better than that of the university program.[7] Anecdotally, this experience has been replicated at the authors' institution. It is not clear, however, if these medical student clerkships improve the number or quality of applicants to the residency program.

Medical students who are considering applying for a surgical residency position can judge their competitiveness by reviewing "Charting Outcomes in the Match," published by The National Residency Matching Program.[10] Surgical residents at independent academic medical centers are demographically different from those at university programs. Applicant characteristics associated with a preference for independent programs include having children, preference for a smaller program, preference for a hospital practice, and having attended a Midwestern medical school. Characteristics of applicants associated with a preference against independent programs include plans for a research year and increased likelihood of pursuing a fellowship.[8]

To further explore applicant demographics and match results at independent surgery programs, Dort and colleagues[11] reviewed information from the Electronic

Residency Application Service. They report that independent programs receive a large number of applications and are selective, interviewing only 12% of the applicants. Of applicants who were interviewed, 81% were ranked for a categorical position. Applicants selected for interview at independent programs predominately graduated from allopathic (MD) medical schools and most had at least 1 academic publication. Applicants were more likely to be ranked if they had scored higher on the United States Medical Licensing Examination (USMLE) Step 1 and Step 2 examinations. Additionally, applicants were more likely to be ranked at by an independent program if they attended medical school in the same region; this was especially true for the Midwest region. This information supports the authors' experience that there is a competitive applicant pool at independent programs and that applicants are motivated to obtain their training geographically close to home.

GRADUATE PERFORMANCE AND OUTCOMES

The ultimate goal of a surgical residency program is to produce surgeons who are competent and compassionate to best meet the needs of their patients and communities. Data regarding outcomes of surgical education at independent programs are somewhat conflicting.

Falcone and Charles[12] reported on the passage rates for the American Board of Surgery Qualifying Examination (QE), a written examination, and the Certifying Examination (CE), an oral examination, for military, university, and community programs for the years 2002 to 2012. They found that community programs had a slightly lower passage rate on both the QE and the CE compared with university and military programs. The overall pass rate for the QE was 85.6%. Community programs had a QE first-time pass rate of 82.6% compared with 86.5% (university) and 93.9% (military). For the CE, community programs had a first-time pass rate of 80.9% compared with 84.8% (university) and 91.0% (military). This finding held when looking at the combined first-time pass rate. Military programs had the highest passage rate. The reasons for the discrepancy between program types are not clear but do not seem related to the size of the program.

Expectedly, there are is a wide variation in the board passage rate among individual programs. These passage rates are available from the American Board of Surgery. Over the most recent 5 years, of 242 general surgery residency programs, there are 8 that have a 100% cumulative first-time pass rate on both the QE and the CE: 4 of these are independent programs, 2 are university programs, and 2 are military programs.[13]

Graduate confidence and competence has become a common subject of discussion in the surgical education community. Because of the early and varied operative experience, independent programs have the reputation of developing surgeons who are confident and competent for practice at the time of graduation. A national survey of 4136 surgical residents revealed that 26% were concerned about their ability to perform procedures by themselves. Training at a community program was independently associated with confidence in operative skills.[14] Residents at university programs were most likely to feel general surgery residency was too long while also expressing a higher rate of concern that they would not feel comfortable operating on their own by the end of their training.[2]

The projected shortage of general surgeons has been widely discussed.[15-17] It is estimated that 50% to 80% of graduates of a general surgery residency program pursue subspecialty fellowship training.[15,16] Independent academic medical centers tend to have faculty members who are broadly trained general surgeons.

Residents are exposed to these role models and practice patterns. After adjusting for hospital size, number of cases, city population, and region, residents who train at community programs pursue a general surgery practice at significantly higher rates than their university counterparts.[15] It is, in part, a result of the selection bias regarding the type of applicant likely to match at a community program. This crucial contribution to the general surgery workforce is also fostered and developed, however, by the general surgeon mentors at independent academic medical centers.

SUMMARY

As discussed previously, there are 3 broad types of surgical residency programs: military, university, and community. Most resident applicants understand university programs because of their experience in medical school. Independent academic medical centers have been involved with surgical resident training for well more than a century. Although there are some unique challenges associated with community programs, there are several benefits of surgical training in the community setting, including a supportive learning environment, early and broad operative exposure, and improved graduate confidence. With the workforce need for general surgeons, independent training programs will continue to play an integral role.

REFERENCES

1. Gupta VF, Jeitmiller RF. Union Memorial Hospital: an insight to the origin of community-based surgical training. J Surg Educ 2008;65(2):162–5.
2. Sullivan MC, Sue G, Bucholz E, et al. Effect of program type on the training experiences of 248 university, community, and US Military-based general surgery residencies. J Am Coll Surg 2012;214(1):53–60.
3. Sullivan MC, Yeo H, Roman SA, et al. Surgical residency and attrition: defining the individual and programmatic factors of trainee losses. J Am Coll Surg 2013; 216(3):461–71.
4. Mahmoud A, Galante J, Wisner D, et al. Small community hospitals programs affiliation with university programs; "lessons learned" in 28-year successful affiliation. J Surg Educ 2013;70(5):636–9.
5. Vaughan A, Welling R, Boberg J. Surgical education in the new millennium: a community hospital perspective. Surg Clin North Am 2004;84:1441–51.
6. McMillen MA. The value of surgical residencies to community teaching hospitals. Arch Surg 1998;133:1039–40.
7. Imperato JC, Rand WM, Grable EE, et al. The role of the community teaching hospital in surgical undergraduate education. Am J Surg 2000;179:150–3.
8. Jarman BT, Joshi ART, Trickey AW, et al. Factors and influences that determine the choices of surgery residency applicants. J Surg Educ 2015. [Epub ahead of print].
9. Johansen K, Heimbach D. So You Want to Be A Surgeon: An Online Guide to Selecting and Matching with the Best Surgery Residency. Available at: https://www. facs.org/education/resources/residency-search. Accessed October 20, 2015.
10. Charting Outcomes in the Match, National Resident Matching Program. Available at: http://www.nrmp.org/nrmpaamc-charting-outcomes-in-the-match/. Accessed September 1, 2015.
11. Dort JM, Trickey AW, Kallies KJ, et al. Applicant characteristics associated with selection for ranking at independent surgery residency programs. J Surg Educ 2015. [Epub ahead of print].

12. Falcone JL, Charles AG. Military and academic programs outperform community programs on the american board of surgery examination. J Surg Educ 2013; 70(5):613–7.
13. Program summary of performance on general surgery exams: 2010-2015. The American Board of Surgery website. Available at: http://www.absurgery.org/default.jsp?prog_passreport. Accessed September 1, 2015.
14. Bucholz EM, Sue GR, Yeo H, et al. Our trainees' confidence – results from a national survey of 4136 US general surgery residents. Arch Surg 2011;146(8): 907–14.
15. Adra SW, Trickey AW, Crosby ME, et al. General surgery vs fellowship: the role of the Independent Academic Medical Center. J Surg Educ 2012;69(2):740–5.
16. Physicians weekly website. Available at: http://www.physiciansweekly.com/general-surgeons-shortage/. Accessed March 26, 2015.
17. Williams TE, Elison EC. Population analysis predicts a future critical shortage of general surgeons. Surg 2008;144(4):548–56.

Index

Note: Page numbers of article titles are in **boldface** type.

Surg Clin N Am 96 (2016) 155–162
http://dx.doi.org/10.1016/S0039-6109(15)00193-0
0039-6109/16/$ – see front matter © 2016 Elsevier Inc. All rights reserved.
surgical.theclinics.com

Moving?

Make sure your subscription moves with you!

To notify us of your new address, find your **Clinics Account Number** (located on your mailing label above your name), and contact customer service at:

Email: journalscustomerservice-usa@elsevier.com

800-654-2452 (subscribers in the U.S. & Canada)
314-447-8871 (subscribers outside of the U.S. & Canada)

Fax number: 314-447-8029

Elsevier Health Sciences Division
Subscription Customer Service
3251 Riverport Lane
Maryland Heights, MO 63043

*To ensure uninterrupted delivery of your subscription, please notify us at least 4 weeks in advance of move.

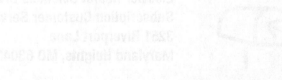

Printed and bound by CPI Group (UK) Ltd, Croydon, CR0 4YY

08/06/2025

01896870-0014